DISC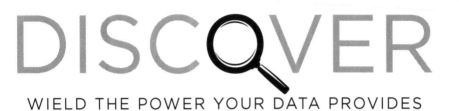VER

WIELD THE POWER YOUR DATA PROVIDES

LIFT

AND BECOME A VICTOR

BECOME

BEYOND THE WEIGHT ROOM

Ayo A. Ajanaku

Re think

First published in Great Britain in 2023
by Rethink Press (www.rethinkpress.com)

Cover image © Shutterstock | anttoniart and Yesaulov Vadym

Jesus Christ is Lord

Contents

Introduction

It is no secret that data has become the single most valuable commodity in the modern business world – and it doesn't look like that will change any time soon. Businesses have used data in enormous quantities to do everything from feeding us mindless forms of entertainment to providing highly specialised medical treatment. From the unproductive to the profitable, data has been used in a variety of ways and has many ecosystems in which it operates. There is, however, one particularly important world to which the application of the data insights have shown to be both inspiring and life changing.

Yours.

If you have a gym membership, whether you use it every day or struggle to go a few times a month, this book is for you. Especially if you have determined to make putting your body through its paces and exerting yourself to train in a way that strengthens you, a regular, ongoing feature of your life.

Every time you do a single pull-up, you are not only strengthening your arms and back, but you are also invigorating the supportive structures involved with the variation of pull-up being performed. This leads to a stronger grip – the kind that allows you to carry home more grocery bags filled with your weekly supermarket delights, without stopping for a rest or needing to quicken your pace. But something even more fascinating happens. Your body and mind begin to adapt to the new stimulus it experiences, creating a healthy and optimal way to manage stress, reduce anxiety, improve confidence, and successfully tackle new challenges.

The kicker is this: unless you know exactly what you are doing and precisely why you are doing it, informed by the data created as you sweat, you are not going to experience the full benefits that weight training can offer. You are training in the metaphorical dark.

In terms of what the best practices are for an individual's training regime, it's a total minefield. Until someone knows what your goals are and how your body responds to a training programme, it will be difficult to keep you consistently committed to a journey for a prolonged period of time and with sustainable outcomes.

In my early days of training, I often had people give me conflicting advice, which has been to my detriment, while they have been able to enjoy the results of their respective training styles. As there is no centralised, data-backed objective knowledge that can guide all individuals on their journey, you will find people doing all kinds of questionable things. You may have seen your fair share of awkward and perhaps amusing gym workouts, performed by people as if they were competing for a place on a gym meme page.

I first picked up a dumbbell when I was twelve and aspiring to fit the 'physically strong' archetype of a man. As I became more aware of my physical capabilities through trial and error in weight training, I found myself achieving far more than I ever dreamed of. For six years, I was one of very few black swimmers at the time competing and winning at national level. Several of my competitors went on to become international swimmers. My relationships with family and friends were filled with the laughter that has you desperately gasping for air but not able to get it together. At fourteen, I earned the respect of coaches at a US basketball camp after coming in as the second most inexperienced player in my age group, with the coaches doubting

I would make any significant progress, and leaving just ten days later as one of the strongest.

At seventeen, my father and I were in a car accident. Our vehicle cannoned into the central reservation before colliding with the hard shoulder barrier on the opposite side where we were hit by another speeding car, which sent us somersaulting down the motorway for 50 metres before coming to a standstill – upside down. Talk about a traumatic experience. This accident should have taken both of our lives. Four months later, I learned how to drive and passed my test first time.

Throughout my adolescence and into adulthood, I have been able to capitalise on the opportunities presented to me and remain resolute through hardships by sustaining a healthy physical outlet so that my relationships wouldn't bear the brunt of my misfortunes. I now work with other people to help them do the same by capturing their data and delivering performance insights that are tailored to their objectives and personal exercise tendencies. This accelerates their progress in achieving not just tangible goals, but also intangible goals, success in which invariably follows what they are seeing in the gym.

If someone were to ask you *why* you train, what answer would you give them? To keep fit and healthy? To look a certain way? To become stronger? While any of these responses may be true, with some introspection you will discover that your answer actually runs much deeper than that. It is a noble thing to want to be healthy and in good shape, but what you are ultimately seeking are the rewards and benefits that come from these things. To be healthy and in good shape is to have improved vigour and vitality, which enables you to experience the fullness of life's pleasures – *that's* the goal.

To achieve greater strength is to experience the benefits of decreased anxiety, more effective management of stress and increased tolerance of pain. This all makes you more formidable and able to valiantly overcome life's hardships.

The point is that the insights you receive from monitoring how your training is going is the bedrock and first building block to living a life that you might otherwise be afraid or doubtful of pursuing. I call this process the 'Cocoon Transformation', and it comprises the four principles detailed in Part Two of this book. It starts with getting crystal clear on your objectives, in knowing what it is you want to get out of training. With the amount of effort, you put in, it is essential to know why you are doing it. This will enable you to pursue a bespoke route to your goals that is safest and most effective for achieving *your* targets – nobody else's.

Next, you will equip yourself with the most potent tools to meet your goals. Artists don't paint with cooking oil, and nor should you be ill-equipped for your efforts in the gym. Here, we'll highlight some often overlooked but fundamental scientific principles about how to drive changes in your body and how you can use this knowledge to your benefit.

This is followed by a framework of thought-processing built to ensure you remain relentlessly consistent in your pursuit, minimising the risk of falling off track. You'll learn how to adopt a fresh and robust perspective when battling against the lack of motivation that inevitably comes for us all at some point.

Lastly, you'll see how this all ties together with the role that artificial intelligence plays in facilitating a process of transformation. The latest and nascent technologies are finding ways into everyday strength training; you can benefit from the insights they provide by making more informed decisions about your health and wellbeing – it's exciting!

Committing yourself to this process will train your mind's eye to become acutely aware of your new experiences in the rebirth phase. At this point, you will be able to live life anew, understanding where your best efforts are focused and persisting in trying to reach your goals. The spoils at this point are not merely physical but volitional, emotional and mental. Although the journey never truly ends, you will know once you have reached this realm of change.

In summary, you first need to equip yourself with twenty-twenty vision to stay in the fight, then you can use AI to keep an up to date blueprint for success for your future reference and replication.

Now let's begin.

PART ONE

THE CASE FOR DATA INSIGHTS

ONE

Data: A Winning Formula At Your Fingertips

In this chapter, we will unpack the mysterious notion of data, explore how it applies to you and understand why it's crucial to achieving your goals in and outside the weight room.

Demystifying data

What comes to mind when you hear the word 'data'? If you are anything like me, you immediately start to think about spreadsheets, computing, transactions and programming languages. This isn't surprising, considering that these are likely to be the contexts in which you have most often heard this term. There are also scores of people out there who are not remotely interested in these fields – you may be one of them.

What often follows, then, is that you instantly switch off when data is brought up in conversation. I don't blame you. Data is so often described and talked about in an abstract way that brings up more questions than it answers, questions like:

- What does this mean?
- Why do I need to know this?
- How does this benefit me?
- What am I expected to do with this information?

These are valid questions to ask, and the answers will enable you to know, understand and use data effectively.

So what actually is data? To put it simply, data is information. That's it. There is nothing inherently mysterious about data. It isn't magic, it isn't elusive, it isn't even clever, in its rawest form – but it is extremely useful. If you know what it is you want and what you are looking for, data will arm you with the most formidable weapon available and can be used to drastically change your circumstances.

Data is truly ubiquitous. You are not only surrounded by it, but you are also producing data every second of every day, in various forms. All of which can inform your thinking and create actionable insights to inspire change and creativity. There will be certain things in your life where data will be logged and recorded every time a particular activity is recognised. For example, when you enter a store and pick up an item that you use your card to pay for, the transaction is recorded in your account and a receipt is generated. When you want to know how much money you have left for the month, or understand where it all went, the spending data that has been collected can be easily used as a point of reference in your banking app. There is no need to commit your balance to memory and then do mental arithmetic every time you make a transaction.

It's all there for you. You can repurpose this data to make it useful to you in myriad ways, whether that be creating a personal budget to facilitate achieving a savings goal, or noticing a pattern of spending that leads you to seek better value for your money.

Despite how integral data is to our lives, there are still many areas in which we don't bother to capture the data that could bring us the greatest advantages. I'm talking about things beyond our bank balance, things that affect our self-perception, the strength of our relationships and how we manage stress and anxiety, to name just a few.

Data and training – the perfect match

When you decide to pack your gym bag, lace up your trainers and head to the gym for a workout, you have decided to do this because it is something you intuitively know is hugely beneficial to you. But you most likely haven't done enough to find out specifically how and why it benefits you. This isn't entirely your fault. There has been little innovation in the gym space compared with other industries, which makes it difficult to know how to use objective and verifiable data to push you in the direction of your goals.

As a teenager, I was fascinated by *Sports Science* on ESPN, which showcased the superhuman feats of several athletes across different sports in a way that was engaging and relatable to real-world experiences. The problem was, as exciting as this was to watch, it was still entertainment. The show featured the world's most elite athletes, at the top of their game, and was directed towards viewers like me: sports enthusiasts, physically active and interested in the data science behind how the human body performs. It was hardly translatable to my life, for personal use – and it wasn't designed to be.

After reaching a certain point, I knew that I had to get more insight on what I was doing in the weight room and the ways in which it was affecting my body. The search for data was on. There is only one way to know how close you are to reaching your exercise targets, and that is to capture information regularly so that you can continually tweak your workout plan so that you can progress as fast as possible.

It baffles me that so many people treat their workout plan as a crystalised set of instructions set in stone, never to be changed. No wonder so many people plateau so quickly. This is not the point of a gym programme. Its purpose is to be a working document to which you can add or take away and that you can adjust based on your ever-changing needs.

Irrespective of whether you love lifting heavy objects in a training centre or competing in a sport that you thoroughly enjoy, you must always pay attention to what the data says about your discipline. If you think you are too clever for that or it's unnecessary, you may find that not only are you not moving towards your goals, but you're in fact regressing away from them.

Do you want that?

SINKING, LOSING AND IGNORING THE DATA

When I started competing as a national swimmer, I knew that it didn't feel 'normal'. This was a massive step up from the Saturday school swimming classes that I had attended from age three.

Everything was so fast paced, so elegant, so intimidating. I wasn't used to this level of intensity, but my parents knew my capabilities and would not let me run away from the challenge. I was always known to be an explosive talent but found that I didn't have the endurance to keep up with the rest of the team during training, which meant I had to work painfully hard to get myself to a sustainable level of fitness.

The crazy thing is that although I was the strongest swimmer in my Saturday classes, I could not then, and still can't now, float on water.

I would watch the other kids lay there effortlessly on the water's surface as if they were enjoying their summer months lying in a hammock on a beach somewhere in the Bahamas. Meanwhile, I was sinking, wondering what on earth I was doing wrong.

My coach would yell 'Just relax, Ayo. Relax!'

'What do you think I'm doing?' I would say to myself quietly, seething with frustration.

This difficulty meant that I had to work harder when it came to swimming, exerting energy both to keep myself afloat and propel myself forward. For this reason, I only enjoyed short bursts of raw power – sprinting.

In my early days of Speedo, White Horse and Kent Junior League meets, I was able to display my explosive power and put on a show for my teammates and coaches, despite being utterly miserable. During this time, I accumulated many trophies and medals, including a club record that stood for six years.

But this was soon to come to a halt. As I grew, my body started to change. I was becoming stronger and heavier. Unlike the graceful displays of our synchro swimmers, I was finding it more difficult to contort my body and manoeuvre my way through water.

I thought that if I was left to train by myself with the help of a trusted coach to oversee me, I could train in a way that was tailored towards power, strength and anaerobic fitness.

I suggested this to my dad, who disagreed. 'You need to listen to your coaches – how can you know better than them?' I knew he wasn't asking me a question. In those fourteen words I was dismissed, and it was never spoken about again.

The results? In a short time, I slowed down. Massively. I stopped winning altogether. No more podium finishes. I was fatigued more easily and regressed in my stroke discipline. It was tough to keep up – I couldn't. Ultimately, I developed a passionate hatred for the sport until, just before I turned sixteen, my parents finally allowed me to quit.

There are a few points in the story above where data insight would have been of great use for comprehending bigger issues and making the required alterations for success. See if you can spot them.

Individualised training is essential if you are seeking the best results.[1] This doesn't apply specifically to swimming – it's the principle that is important, and this applies to weight training in the same way it does to every other physical activity.

The law of marginal gains

When you wish to make seismic improvements in your training, you may be fooled into thinking that this requires you to go out and stock up on protein, creatine, branched-chain amino acids (BCAAs), pre-workout glutamine and eggs. . . all at the same time. Then you might think some new gear wouldn't go amiss, so add it to your shopping basket. Logic will then dictate to you that, as you now have everything you need, you should start using it religiously because therein lies the key to greater gains or faster recovery.

Let's slow down for a minute and think reasonably about this. I'm not saying there is anything particularly wrong with any of these things, or that you should avoid using them. Not at all. I am saying, though, that it's easy to get led down a rabbit hole and allow distractions to divert your attention away from the process that delivers the results you desperately want to see.

The law of marginal gains holds that tiny yet significant improvements will cumulatively lead to an enormous overall result. These marginal gains can often be found in the types of changes to your training plan that you are likely to ignore or neglect. This is a grave error – your success lies within those small but frequent modifications. They usually don't appear exciting or ground-breaking, or even entirely relevant at times. Don't let this fool you. You should see each little change as one piece of a larger puzzle, without which you will not be able to fully realise your vision and goals.

As you make the journey to the realm of high performance, there are a host of other characteristics and micro-benefits of the law of marginal gains that will help you get there. A key one is a sustainable level of development.

One of the things that keeps people stuck in a rut when it comes to progress is the difficulty of making colossal alterations to match their ambitions, only for them to fall by the wayside and be given up entirely later on. As lofty and well intentioned as your aims may be, emulating this style of 'improvement' is unsustainable and will leave you disheartened.

The idea behind marginal gains is that, as you are only making incremental changes to your workout programme, they are more likely to pass through practically undetected, which means sticking to your schedule is much easier to sustain.[2] For instance, presume for a moment that you want to increase your muscle mass and usually take enough rest between sets to feel good enough to repeat the set successfully. Let's assume the time between sets averages four or five minutes as you sit there on TikTok or Instagram scrolling away while the irritated man next to you wonders when you'll finally be done with the machine.

As your goal here is muscle mass and not necessarily muscle strength, you should ditch the phone and make an incremental improvement to your rest time. Several studies have indicated that the optimal rest time when working on muscle mass is between thirty and ninety seconds.[3] The reason for this is because, in this instance, you are trying to overload your muscles and stimulate the muscle fibres by causing them temporary trauma. This is an example of a small change with a big outcome – and that's just one.

THE DOMINANCE OF BRITISH CYCLING

Historically, British cycling was not a sport in which the nation could boast dominance on the world stage.[4]

Although there had been some modest successes up until the end of the twentieth century, there certainly wasn't anything to suggest it was time to brace ourselves for a global change in the way we perceived British cycling.

For decades at a time, there were no celebrations to be had for World Championship and Olympic medallists, leaving many competitors and aspiring cyclists discouraged and spiritless. That is, until 2002, when Dave Brailsford was appointed Performance Director of British Cycling. Although the concept of marginal gains had been around for many decades, it was his under his supervision of the programme, and in light of the subsequent results, that it rose to prominence.

Ahead of the London 2012 Olympics, the task was to optimise key factors such as the aerodynamics of the cyclist and bike, the ergonomics of the seat, the grip of the tyres and countless other minute changes.

This optimisation persisted into other, less obvious areas too. The team's strategists implemented changes to things like the massage gels and pillows that were used by the cyclists, along with practising the best methods of hand washing to prevent infection.

These aggregated changes had lasting and world-class effects. During the London 2012 Olympics, Britain established itself as the leading authority in world cycling when the team achieved eight gold medals – the most of any country competing in the sport.

Many of you will not have the resources and expertise needed to make hundreds of tiny changes in order to increase your performance and move the needle closer to your goals. That's fine. Unless you are competing at an elite level, which mandates you to use every legal advantage you can get your hands on to win, you won't need all that extra help.

The key takeaway is this: start gathering some workout data and use it to examine your workout activity. Rigorously scrutinise a few of the practices you're used to doing, then ask one of the personal trainers in your gym if they would be happy to give you their professional opinion on what they think might be holding you back.

The wider implications for you

Although the law of marginal gains is widely applied in the sporting world, the benefits have far-reaching implications. Being able to identify areas of deficiency or inefficiency that impede your ability to meet your objectives in the weight room will teach you how to evaluate your circumstances and make good judgements beyond that.

Consider for a moment that you have loaded up the barbell for your bench press and, as you reach the halfway point of your third set, you feel an unfamiliar strain in the left side of your chest. You don't think much of it and persist with another rep until you feel the strain become a little tighter. Now you're faced with two options:

1. Stop because you don't want to risk injury.

2. Continue because you want to finish the set.

You decide to stop. As determined a person you are, you're also sensible and want to live to train another day. By making this decision, not only have you potentially avoided serious injury, you have also sharpened your risk assessment skills. There will be times when you'll be faced with a circumstance for which your calculation of risk versus reward will compel you to be risk-seeking and grab an opportunity with both hands. On other occasions, risk aversion will be the order of the day. This assessment trains your mind's eye to tread carefully in pursuit of both preservation and prosperity. As I said, this has far-reaching consequences. It may be that you've been putting off that prostate exam for a bit too long. In which case, you decide it's high time to pick up the phone and schedule the appointment.

Just as there is a real practical benefit of marginal gains, there can also be serious consequences for those who wish to ignore it. One of the reasons why our starting point is data related to weight-training activity is because there is something innately revealing about being able to delineate where your body is right now from its data. It's personal. From this, deeper external patterns are also discovered.

A few years ago, I remember making a derisive comment about my brother's temporary obsession with the cleanliness and appearance of his teeth. He, being interested in property, replied, 'If I can't even be trusted to take care of my teeth, how is someone going to trust me with their property?' As funny as I found this, I had nothing in response. His perspective that taking his appearance seriously would help get from where he was to where he wanted to be is a healthy one.

The world is moving at a blistering pace and if you fail to adhere to principles that position you for success then, although you will still be moving, you will despair when you realise you've been moving in the wrong direction. Then, all those things you said you didn't want (only you know what they are) will slowly start creeping into your life. Determine right now that this won't be you.

Avoid pitfalls through team accountability

Before we take a closer look at the ideas behind tailoring our training to our unique physiological characteristics, let's talk about how to avoid the common pitfall of giving up before you've even started.

As with any endeavour worth pursuing, you'll need not only to arm yourself with the right knowledge but also to surround yourself with the right people, those who will drive you forward towards your vision. A lot of keen and would-be gym-goers think that it's necessary to search high and low to find these people, but that isn't necessarily the case. Heading to the gym with your friends who already go, having regular conversations with a few personal trainers, or getting involved in an online community as an active member are all ways to become enmeshed in the training ecosystem of accountability. As long as you do this in a consistent and incremental way, you'll find that you have a sustainable means to keep on track as well as opening yourself up to immense opportunities for learning. This will work to motivate you when distractions or laziness try to pull you off course.

This has become so natural to me that, after more than a few days of inactivity, I start to become a restless grouch with no desire to apply myself to work or anything else. It's also exemplified in the inspirational story of KC.

FRIEND OF THE GYM

I have met few people who are as vibrant as KC Bulaon. She is a prime example of what it looks like to be a high-spirited individual. KC always seemed to have the inner workings of an influential ally, but strength training was the key that enabled her to realise her potential.

For several years in her late teens and early twenties, KC was active in trying various forms of exercise to stay healthy and look better while enjoying the thrill of a new challenge. Nothing clicked until, at the age of twenty-one, she went to Australia for a year and met a personal trainer who encouraged her to try lifting. KC had free access to a gym and all the time she could ask for to train, but she was still shy and felt like she didn't know what she was supposed to be doing.

Fast forward a year and when KC returned to London she started to strength train with two of her male friends. This was a major inflection point on her journey. KC would do German Volume Training (an intense type of strength training) three times a week and loved the feeling her body experienced after undergoing such gruelling activity – but perhaps the thing that KC loved most was that she got to spend quality time with her friends doing something productive. Under the guidance of a new personal trainer, KC became technically competent and started to notice a significant improvement in her strength.

Since her return to London, KC has built many strong relationships through going to the gym and training with men and women alike. She believes that strength training matched her energy and desire to achieve her loftiest goals – beautiful.

After one training session she was by the gym lockers when two women commented on her strength and confidence in using an area that was intimidating to them – the weights area. One of the women was adamant that she couldn't use the space because it was 'too scary'. KC reassured the woman that strength training areas are not just for men. KC invited the woman to train together with her and meet the other people KC had befriended who used the space. Within a few months, KC's new friend had learned a huge amount from her and was deadlifting more than KC was. Together, they enjoyed almost three consistent years of accountability as training partners.

Whether it is pushing herself to the outer limits of her capabilities or helping a stranger do the same, KC always seems to be asking the same question: how does the way I apply myself in the gym make me a better and more confident friend? One thing is for sure: the strength of her relationships shows she already knows the answer.

Summary

You now know what data is and how integral it is to your objectives. Data is information that you gain from learning, research and experience. When it's used effectively, it gives you an unmatched edge and propels you towards achieving your goals. Ignore it, and you will be leaving piles of untapped potential undiscovered.

FOUR

Get Clear On Your Objectives

In this chapter, we will learn how to use your curated data and information to set powerful objectives in the weight room, objectives that transcend this context and have a ripple effect on your life outside the gym. You need to be crystal clear in your mind about your objectives before you begin strength training, but there is something else you need to engage in first.

Identify your pain points

Any individual, anywhere on earth who picks up a weight to train is not doing it simply to achieve a physical goal. The reason always runs deeper than that. You might be training so that you have a healthy outlet to cope with a stress-inducing lifestyle. Perhaps you're training because you're looking for a new partner and want to be in the best shape possible to build your confidence and self-esteem. It could be that strength training helps you to feel safer in your everyday life, particularly if there's a chance you may face dangerous situations. Whatever the reason for training, it can always be traced back to something deeply personal to you. It's important you identify and keep focus on what this is as it will anchor your efforts and give purpose to your pursuit.

With this in mind, take stock of all of the pain points you're currently experiencing in your life to which *you* are a contributor. Sometimes we can encounter unfortunate circumstances or endure a run of bad luck, but these things on their own are not typically sufficient to keep someone down long-term. More often than not, we harm our own chances of reaching our aspirations by doing things we know we shouldn't, and not doing the things we know we need to do to get where we want to be. These behaviours lead to a self-inflicted kind of pain point.

Write down some examples of these pain points for you – somewhere, anywhere – it will help to organise your thoughts. Think about them as often as you can. I can't understand why people choose to bury their heads in the sand and are happy pretending everything is hunky dory when they know deep down it isn't. You must face your problems and pain head on;

instead of denying, embrace them and wrap your mind around them. Let them become familiar to you. This has nothing to do with having a poor attitude or a negative perception of yourself, but it does have everything to do with adding a pound of realism and recognising how you are self-sabotaging. Once you know this, you will be in a position to change it. It's about being self-aware.

You might not think this has anything to do with weight training, but it does. By the end of this book, you will understand how this picture comes together. Strength training is not the goal for most people, but rather the vehicle that takes them to their true goal. There's no way you would be engaged in such strenuous activity if you were content to gain weight and slip into an unhealthy lifestyle. If you were happy to do that, you wouldn't be reading this book.

Something else that can be uncomfortable, but necessary, to think about are the reasons you are exhibiting the behaviours you've identified as causing your pain points. When you do this, try not to view circumstances or the behaviour of others as excuses for your shortcomings. You will never grow that way. For example, if you are short-tempered with your loved ones then instead of rationalising it by insisting that they're the ones who are aggravating you (something outside of your control), be honest with yourself and admit that you could work on improving your patience (something within your control).

Your strength training will help you cultivate this way of thinking if you're conscious of it. Instead of looking for excuses, you will begin to take ownership of your circumstances in the same way that you take ownership of your body through your weight training and strength goals. As you arm yourself with the right tools to grow in physical strength, so must you apply the same principles in gathering as much information as you can about your behaviours, attitudes and tendencies to grow in other areas too. Once you've fully understood precisely how you are holding yourself back, you will be better for it and can start working on how to move forward.

Take note of your aspirations

After you've considered your pain points and what's driving them, the next thing to meditate on and write down is your immediate aspirations. Put these in places that you know you'll see regularly. This could be in a notes app on your phone, images on your desktop background, or musings on your bathroom mirror. You won't always be consciously reading what you've written every time your eyes fall on these reminders, but you will be subconsciously feeding your desires to drive action that will aid you in the pursuit of these aspirations.

Figuring out what these immediate aspirations are is a simple task. They will usually be the antonym of your current pain points, to which you are a major or the sole contributor, as we've already mentioned. It is worth re-emphasising that this will require a degree of honesty that you may normally be uncomfortable with. To have aspirations that you have not previously been on the road to fulfilling is to acknowledge the part you have played in the delay to achieving them. Getting clear on your objectives is a prerequisite for success and doing so early will avoid stagnation further down the line.

As well as having reminders of your aspirations written in places you'll see regularly, make an active effort to embrace them and think about them often. Never underestimate the power of your thoughts. You won't change your life with a few days of mere 'positive thinking', but remarkable things will happen if you make a habit of directing your thoughts towards personal aspirations that are meaningful to you and arise from a genuine pain. Actively embracing these thoughts has a cumulative effect on what you decide to do and how you feel about your circumstances, sharpening your focus.

Whether your goals are to shift some unwanted pounds or increase your personal bests, what we've discussed so far will help you build a formidable training plan and keep your focus on the right side of the road as you hit your milestones. There are some skills that you will have already acquired in this endeavour; these are easy to overlook, but you should fully appreciate them. When you build and execute a training programme, you are exercising patience and demonstrating a commitment to meeting your goals and objectives. When you exercise a virtue, it grows. These skills aren't limited to the weight room; they are characteristics that filter through into all you do in life. The patience that you build in sticking with a training schedule that you're not seeing instant results from will be the same patience that you will need to tactfully handle conflict resolution. You might apply it differently, but the virtue is the same.

You will know from experience that you cannot rush the natural process of strength gain, so you will become acutely aware that neither can you rush or force an amicable reconciliation. You can only use the tools you have available to you to try and bring about the desired result. Luckily for you, your results are rooted in science and don't involve the opinions of others. Likewise, when you decide to skip training for no good reason, or fail to honour your commitment to your physical goals, you are further ingraining negative traits such as indolence or irresponsibility, which will inevitably carry through to other areas of your life.

In the pursuit of your strength and training goals, you will acquire and nurture the positive virtues that will work in your favour and help you to achieve the wider aspirations you wrote down earlier.

DOUBTER TO CHALLENGE-SEEKER

I would be doing you a disservice if I didn't include in this book the experiences of a friend of mine, Michele Rosso. Michele wasn't the most active teenager, initially. In fact, he was seriously overweight, which led to him being bullied by his peers. Fortunately, he learned not to internalise any acerbic remarks but knew he wanted to do something about it. When he was sixteen, he decided to lose the weight and get in shape.

Every day for two months, when he felt hungry he would grab his bike and ride for miles, instead of eating. He managed to lose 30kg in those two months, but he'd done it in the worst possible way and suffered many avoidable health issues as a result.

After high school, Michele worked in a factory in a job he did not enjoy. He told me about the pressure, tough physical demands, few rest breaks, constant monitoring and no communication with his fellow workers. It was a mentally suffocating experience for him and he hated it with every fibre of his being. The few minutes he sat in the staff room before his shift was punctuated by a familiar alarm that sent dread through Michele's body, a stark warning that his ten-hour shift was about to begin.

During this time, Michele joined an independent gym that he frequented often. It became the sanctuary he needed to endure his factory work. Here, he met a guy who introduced him to StrongFirst, a global provider of strength education. To pass the course, Michele needed to complete both a physical and a theoretical test. Because he wanted to become exceptional in his field, he also pursued a degree in exercise science alongside his StrongFirst training course.

He also took a new job, in a restaurant, which meant he was often coming home at 3am to train and study for his tests. I think it's fair to say his hands were full.

Michele had never enjoyed studying up to this point and wasn't particularly good at it. He even doubted whether it was worth his efforts, but after a conversation with a Master's graduate at his gym, he decided to give it his best shot. So high were the odds stacked against him that his own friends had a bet among themselves that Michele would fail his first exam and then end up quitting university.

It was during this pivotal time in his life that the penny dropped for Michele. He was starting to realise the positive impact training was having on achieving his personal goals, and he was hooked. His fierce determination grew and his resolve was strengthening with every battle that came to test him. Michele successfully completed the StrongFirst training course and, in 2022, he was one of just 101 people to have ever successfully completed the Beast Tamer challenge in the StrongFirst programme.

Today, his physique is near perfect and his outlook on life is supremely positive. He has used his experience and knowledge to help hundreds of people get similar results.

Oh, and the bet that Michele's friends had? That didn't turn out too well for them. The hours and effort Michele put in paid off, he passed his first exam the first time around and went on to complete his Bachelor's degree in exercise science. This was one of his proudest achievements, because of what he had to overcome to get there, and he told me, 'I attribute that achievement, and many others like it, to the gym.'

Muscle building, fat loss and strength training

If you've decided that your goal is to become a sculpted work of art, then that will affect how you train. With hypertrophy as the primary goal and strength development as the secondary goal, there are particular elements that you should incorporate into your training to accelerate your progress. Different goals necessitate different training approaches. The issue for most is that they have no idea what these differences are and so decide to pick up a weight and train in an unstructured way.

The average person has a general understanding that there is a correlation between muscle size and strength. I mean, when have you ever seen a skinny guy deadlift 200kg? But the degree of this correlation isn't well understood. Several studies have explored this, with interesting results. Generally, muscle activation occurs to a greater degree in smaller muscles than in larger ones. Muscle activation is simply how well your mind can instruct a particular muscle to switch on and work; the stronger this connection, the stronger the activation. This typically leads to a higher force production, which equates to more strength.

When it comes to simply building muscle, you want to focus on your range of motion, also referred to as the length-tension curve, which is more important for some muscle groups than others where the improvements seen from a fuller range of motion are negligible.[12] An example can be found in the studies showing that deep squats that exhibit a full range of motion induce higher quad growth than squats done with a partial range of motion.[13] Whereas the same full range of motion principle applied to the bicep curl turns out to be inconsequential relative to a partial range of motion.[14]

When people speak about their enthusiasm (or lack thereof) for their mission to lose weight, what they're usually expressing is a desire to lose fat. As muscle is denser than fat, this means many people don't believe that you can lose fat and gain or maintain muscle at the same time, which is what we refer to as body recomposition, causing them a dilemma. However, several studies have provided evidence that it is possible.[15] One of the key reasons why building muscle through strength training is so appealing is because bigger muscles need more energy, which increases your metabolism, which in turn leads to more calories being burned – reducing the volume of fat in your body.

There are some things you can do to help you on your way to experiencing body recomposition:[16]

- The generally accepted rule is to consume at least 2.2g of protein per 1kg of bodyweight (1g/lb), as you need a high protein intake to gain muscle.

- Train by consistently lifting heavy weights – you want to give your body a mechanical stimulus that is strong enough to force it to maintain muscle.

- Don't forget to rest. The optimal amount of sleep time every twenty-four hours should be about eight hours, which is a third of your day. This may not be easy to achieve, but you need to make sure you compensate for any sleep deprivation during the day where possible for maximal results.

Managing stress

Another reason why you may have chosen to weight train is because you either live a hectic life or have enough stress-inducing moments to warrant finding a healthy outlet for all that pent up tension. The gym is used as a way to cope with the fast-paced and unpredictable nature of life by millions of people around the world.

It's often said that human beings do not like change, and even avoid it. People are creatures of habit and do not generally like things interfering with their regular routines of life. In an era where change is happening at an unprecedented rate, going to the gym regularly is a physical activity that many find comfort in, but its benefits can be even greater than that. When I was studying for my accounting finals, my tutor and friend, Sean Purcell, told the class, 'The only real way to relieve stress is to force it out at the gym.' I understood straight away what he was alluding to because I had been experiencing it for years. What I came to understand better, though, was the science behind that statement. In 2017, a meta-analytical study concluded that weight training significantly improved anxiety symptoms among both healthy participants and participants with physical or mental illness.[17] Not marginally, but *significantly* improved symptoms.

Before we move on to talk about equipping yourself for battle, let me level with you once again and tell you that your deepest and most sincere goals are not related to a number on the scale, or the size of the weight pushed in the gym. What matters most to you will go far deeper than anything you can physically achieve through effort and willpower. I don't know what that is for you, but you will be able to discover it with a little thought and introspection.

Although your achievements are not necessarily the prize, they will help you get closer to realising your desires. Strength training is the vehicle we're travelling in, and the cumulative effects of this engagement have been shown to have transformative effects in a variety of areas, from cognitive ability to injury prevention. For example, your bone density decreases significantly as you age. It becomes brittle and weak, so falls become more serious and hip replacements more likely. Strength training does a magnificent job of increasing bone density and those who engage it, even in old age, aren't as at risk from accidental falls as people who don't.

Aside from the physical benefits associated with strength training, you are using one of the most robust and proven ways to augment the quality of intangibles such as accountability, moderation and reliability, to name a few. Having both physical and psychological advantages on your side will inspire and compel you to do the things that push you towards living more purposefully and prioritising the things that matter most to you. Perhaps you haven't previously seen it this way and so have allowed a lot of your efforts to be wasted.

Moving forward, it is important you don't neglect the steps along the way while keeping the bigger picture in mind, while also remembering that the whole process is underpinned by data. The big picture, broken down into steps, looks like this:

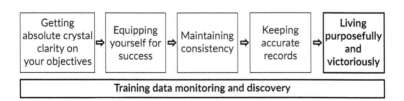

| Getting absolute crystal clarity on your objectives | ⇨ | Equipping yourself for success | ⇨ | Maintaining consistency | ⇨ | Keeping accurate records | ⇨ | Living purposefully and victoriously |

| Training data monitoring and discovery |

DIESEL THE STRONGMAN

I have a friend who I call Diesel, not only because he is a walking vessel of power, but because his unmistakable passion for training and competing are the engine behind his endowed stature. Other people know him as Dan Thomas.

At age fourteen months, his mum saw him take his first steps after he'd crawled into the kitchen only to pull himself up on his little chair, pick it up and *walk out* with it.

Dan has always been naturally stronger than his peers. At eleven he was helping his dad push start his Vauxhall Estate on cold mornings and later moving the class anvil to his workstation during metal work when his teacher had left the room.

As mighty as this sounds, Dan was also being bullied for his weight. His self-esteem was dissolving but he would later come to view this as a momentous season in his life. At thirteen, he was lifting the weights his parents bought him for his birthday and soon after he was even bigger and stronger than all the bullies – he was also in much better shape. The bullying stopped, but his journey was just beginning.

After his parents divorced when he was a teenager, Dan struggled. He wasn't training like he should and became estranged from his dad. At twenty, he turned to alcohol to numb his pain and frustrations.

But one day in his mid-twenties, everything changed. Dan had won a cocktail-making competition and had his picture published in a magazine. He was mortified at the person staring back at him – who he saw in the picture was not the same person he saw in the mirror. Dan stopped drinking altogether for six months and started training again. Around this time he also started armwrestling competitively. He had taken what was previously the crutch of strength training and turned it into a sword to kill his vices and self-doubts.

The strength he developed in his arms, back, forearms and wrists was demonstrated in the five consecutive years that he finished in the top three positions at the British Armwrestling Championships. He also competed in two World Championships.

After he wisely decided to stop competing following a horrible injury sustained during one of his competitions, Strongman was next on Dan's agenda. If there's anyone who keeps detailed training and lifestyle notes – it's Diesel Thomas. He applied his studious mind and attentive eye to identifying patterns in his workout data, which was instrumental to his many achievements. Here are a few:

- Won his first Strongman competition in 2016
- Placed top three in his next eight competitions
- Placed sixth in Southern England's Strongest Man
- Qualified for England's Strongest Man
- Won London's Strongest Master
- Placed fifth in the European Championships held by Official Strongman Games
- Recorded the longest time for the front hold event, across all weight classes
- Placed sixteenth in the World Championships held by Official Strongman Games

What makes these achievements even more impressive is that Dan accomplished them with numerous physiological conditions that should have made such things impossible.

Reflecting on his journey, he told me, 'If lockdown had happened to me when I was twenty-four, I'd have been dead in three months. . . Lifting and competing literally saved my life [and] gave me discipline over alcohol. That discipline has made me a better coach and professional.'

Dan is a warm-hearted giant who understands the benefits of strength training more than most. Whether their goals are to live longer, be fit enough to run around after their kids or to improve their mental health by having a positive outlet for stress, Dan passes on his knowledge to his clients so that they too can have the best quality of life available to them – *that* is what this is all about.

Summary

You now know that the most powerful and dynamic way to set your strength-training objectives is by linking them to your pain points and deeper aspirations. After this, you'll have laid the foundation to become intensely focused on how to build strength while simultaneously losing fat. This journey can seem like a stressful one at times, so it's important to maintain an appropriate stress management perspective.

FIVE
The Right Tools

In this chapter, you will learn about some of the more technical aspects of the physiological changes your body will undergo during training and some principles to keep your body functioning optimally.

Body recomposition

There are instances, which might be familiar to you, where an avid and seemingly committed gym-goer consistently spends their hard-earned money on a gym membership and puts in consistent and active effort, only to fail to see any notable results. Meanwhile, the newbie who joined a few months ago is making leaps and bounds in their training results. Why? Is it because there are what people call 'non-responders' to exercise? Or is it because there are a handful of people in every district who have magic genes? The available evidence doesn't support either of these claims. It is unlikely that global non-responders to exercise exist; instead, a more individually focused approach to exercise prescription is advised to overcome any apparent non-responsiveness.[18]

The issue for our stagnating friend is more likely a lack of knowledge, or they are adopting a training programme that is not suited to their genetic makeup in terms of intensity, volume or modality. This can (and should) be changed to a more favourable, tailored approach.

When it comes to body recomposition, there is a prolific school of thought that holds that it only happens to those who are completely new to strength training or those who are severely overweight. The idea that relatively well-trained individuals who are no strangers to the gym are not able to gain muscle mass while simultaneously losing fat has been disproven by several studies.[19] If this is a goal of yours, then it is most certainly possible, but it's not enough to put in the work in the gym without giving the same attention to your diet. Diet is one of the key contributors to body recomposition, so much so that it has been shown to have an influence as a standalone measure.[20] When you combine the right diet with strength training, the results have the potential to be huge.

Delving into the nuances of nutrition and how it serves your physical transformation purposes is outside the scope of this book, but there are some great practical books that make it easy to reorient your diet to serve this objective.[21] Alternatively, if you have access to a nutritionist they will have a wealth of knowledge and be able to provide evidence-based nutritional strategies for a healthy diet that facilitates a decrease in fat mass. The model example would be the Mediterranean diet, which is widely recommended due to it being one of the most balanced and healthy diets for promoting cardiovascular and metabolic health.[22]

Strength and muscle growth – tension

An increase in your gym knowledge will not always lead to increased strength. Research has found that motivation, accountability and knowledge of effective weight-training techniques are all required for enhanced progress.[23] Accountability will help you stay on track, whether you enjoy what you're doing or not, and knowledge of effective training techniques will help you to achieve your goals, which will be a powerful source of motivation.

Progressive overload is a commonly used but largely misunderstood term. You most probably know how important volume is for muscle growth and strength, which is commonly calculated as reps × weight × sets = total weight. While you may obsess over the details for your lifts, your muscles only really register one thing – *tension*. They're not registering how much weight you're lifting or how many reps you're performing. Of course, adding weight and increasing the number of reps is an effective way to increase tension and promote muscle growth, but it isn't always the best way. It certainly isn't the only way, but it is the most common.

You can't add weight and reps forever; we are all limited by our human capabilities. Ignoring this and trying to push yourself to extremes will only cause your form to deteriorate and become dangerous. This means that you're actually reducing the tension stimulation you're applying to your target muscle, which makes this an exercise in futility.

Tension stimulation is arguably the most important factor as far as your training is concerned because it's what determines muscle growth and strength and can be achieved at any weight, providing you train within three to five repetitions of failure.[24] The evidence for this is compelling; studies have shown no notable difference in muscle volume between subjects who trained at 30% of their one-rep max (1RM) and those who trained at 90% of their 1RM.[25]

Having said that, we also want to consider how a desire to increase strength gains influences our training exercises. If strength is the goal, then the data suggests that lifting at weights around 80% of your 1RM is optimal for maximising muscle activation.[26]

However, it's also important to consider that your 1RM can fluctuate by up to 18% on any given day as a result of other things going on in your life – you'll surely have noticed that some days you feel stronger and more energised than others.[27] Nonetheless, using this measure when lifting weights in general means that your contraction velocity is slower, which results in even greater tension stimulation of the muscles.

Incorporating progressive overload into your training will lead to strength and muscle gains you can be proud of. In summary, if you want to stimulate maximum muscle strength and growth, you're going to have to lift some heavy weights and lift them close to failure. This is exemplified in the story of Rai.

THE WORDS OF A CHAMPION

In sixth form, Rai would watch one of his schoolteachers train inexperienced boys in rowing; many of these boys would later become Olympians. The weight equipment caught his fancy and when Rai asked if he could be allowed to use it, the teacher-coach obliged.

After only a few months, Rai noticed massive performance changes when he played football. He was solid on the ball, he was agile, graceful and his power was mounting. For full disclosure, it must be admitted that Rai is genetically gifted, but this doesn't mean that hard work wasn't an indispensable part of the equation.

He carried on lifting weights while playing football and was selected to play for Middlesex County Schools after dominating the trials and impressively scoring from the halfway line, which doesn't happen every day.

It wasn't until after he left school that Rai joined the gym to take his weight training more seriously. At twenty-one, after a year of training, he competed in his first bodybuilding competition – UKBFF Stars of Tomorrow.

After this, all Rai wanted was to be big. He knew that strength would come with it, but his primary motivation was to become intimidating enough to deter the racist and tyrannical behaviour of the National Front supporters in his area, who were on the rise at the time.

By his mid-twenties, he'd got exactly what he wanted. In his words, he became a 'human dustbin', finishing off his friends' meals and eating everything and anything he could. He was also training like he was about to go to war in a zombie apocalypse.

The result? Rai became 19.5 stone of mass.

By this point, you can probably guess what kind of racial abuse he would have shouted at him in the street – *nothing*. In fact, people who didn't know Rai were terrified of him, often crossing the road upon seeing him walking towards them. He was so big that, on a trip to Mumbai for a friend's wedding, he was followed on the beach by an entourage of twenty people taking pictures of him.

One day, he gets a call from a close friend who had opened his own gym. 'Isn't it time you compete again?' Rai agreed but he'd left it late; he had two months to get his physique chiselled and in proper condition for the qualifying show for the EFBB British Bodybuilding Championships. They were a painful two months;

sacrifices were made, with the mentality that he had to work harder than anyone else. The day of the qualifying show rolls around and the judges knew who the winner was as soon as Rai walked onto the stage.

The EFBB British Championships were just two weeks later and the same thing happened. The winner was clear from the outset and the sold-out theatre erupted in ferocious applause when first place was awarded to Rai Garcia-Singh.

These achievements showed Rai that he could do more than he thought he was capable of, a lesson he applies to his everyday life. Through his strength training, he has made friends for life, featured in *The Fifth Element*, and worked with high-powered people who also want to be strong and fit because, as he says, 'Strength training is the fountain of youth.'

Rest and recovery

We've spoken a lot about activity, but not enough yet about rest. There are two considerations here, both signs that you're not prioritising rest:

1. Overreaching

2. Overtraining

Overreaching comes first and can be defined as 'muscle soreness above and beyond what you typically experience that occurs when you don't sufficiently recover between workouts'.[28] This is what you might experience after several consecutive days of sustained high-intensity or volume training. If you decide to ignore this level of muscle soreness and continue training, you'll move into a state of overtraining, which is much worse. While overreaching can be easily reversed with a few days of rest, overtraining does more damage to the body and is more difficult to overcome, with full recovery requiring several weeks or even months of rest. Overtraining is more likely when there are other stressors in your life, for example a stressful job, constant travelling or not getting adequate sleep.

Remember that mental wellness, healthy sleep and good nutrition are all critically important for your training regime for you to experience its full benefits. No matter your goals in the weight room, your gains are always made outside the gym while your body is resting and recovering. As well as soreness and decreased performance, if you're starting to feel increased tension such as anger, confusion and irritability, it could be a sign that you need to slow down and make some changes. That's not the direction our training is supposed to be taking us in.

Here are three simple things that you can do to avoid the negative effects of overtraining.

1. Sleep

The Sleep Foundation recommends that, for most adults, at least seven hours of sleep every night is needed to maintain healthy cognitive and behavioural function.[29] Less sleep may feel normal to you, but the likelihood is that your body has developed a tolerance to sleep deprivation. This isn't a good thing and it contributes to higher risk of illness in the future. In addition, it's during the physically restorative stage of sleep, called 'slow-wave' sleep, that 95% of growth hormones are released; this aids muscle recovery and eases aches and pains sustained during training.[30]

2. Hydration

Keeping hydrated is essential for your muscles to remain strong and energised. When you sweat, your body loses lots of electrolytes, which are needed for the muscles to function efficiently. Making sure that you are hydrated will promote healthy blood flow; this increases the supply of oxygen to the brain and muscles, which will mitigate fatigue. If you've ever had a blood test, you will recall the practitioner telling you to make sure you drink plenty of water beforehand, for exactly this reason.

3. Nutrition

You need to put into your body what you hope to get out of it. This will be difficult for some people and easier for others, but you must make an active effort to ensure that your caloric intake is sensible for your level of activity and that the nutritional value of the food you eat reflects your goals.

Neglecting nutrition but perfecting sleep and hydration could still have you feeling fatigued and performing poorly. All three factors work together and are essential fuel allowing your strength-training vehicle to carry you to the destination you want to reach.

'NOT LIKE THIS!'

In the first few months after I picked up Brazilian Jiu-Jitsu (BJJ), I was making immense progress. My coach was one of the most unassuming and humblest people you could ever meet, but I knew the dangers that could befall anyone who made the mistake of seeing him as an easy target. He was a weapon. Not only had he been a black belt for years before he'd even turned thirty, but he'd also won all his professional mixed martial arts (MMA) fights.

I was under great guidance, and it showed.

I had an unfair advantage among the rest of the class. I was much stronger than they were – and they knew it. It was for this reason that I was able to spar competitively with anyone in my gym, irrespective of the colour of their belt.

I remember sparring with a guy called Joker who was not only more experienced than me in BJJ but also had a long and passionate run in MMA. Not long into our sparring session, he'd put himself in a beautiful position primed to use all his force to crank my right arm into an arm-bar submission. He couldn't.

'What kind of superhuman strength is this?' he remarked.

It wasn't because I was particularly good at BJJ at the time that he was unable to make me submit at that point, he was still a far technically superior fighter to me. I was just much stronger.

A guy called Casiano, an even more experienced fighter than Joker, absolutely detested sparring with me. He said I was dangerous and that I didn't know Jiu-Jitsu. I couldn't believe this guy. There was one session where the coach put us together to fight. I was reluctant due to his previous complaints about my dominant and 'dangerous' fighting style, but I acquiesced. After a couple of minutes, I had him in some discomfort – that's when the lecture began.

'Not like this! You don't learn anything today!' He was incensed. I apologised but said nothing more in response. He begrudgingly finished the fight with me, although I toned it way down.

Once we were done, I went straight to the bench to sit and drink some water while I thought about what he said, staring blindly into the mats. 'Am I really that indiscriminate in my techniques? Why am I not picking up what I've been learning?' A few seconds had passed when I saw my coach walking in my direction. Unbeknownst to me, he had seen and heard everything.

He bent over and leaned into me, as if to tell me something important. He said in a firm but calm voice, 'Do not listen to this bulls**t. Your strength is your gift and it is what makes you. He doesn't like that – go easy on him.'

When people resent you for the things you've worked hard to achieve, it isn't a nice feeling, but that comment from my coach was exactly what I needed in that moment.

The reason my sparring style was what it was is that I needed to get the job done quickly – my fast-twitch muscle fibres would fatigue quickly, which meant I struggled to go the distance and so had my ass whooped more times than I'd like to remember.

It was a rude awakening that I needed to adjust my training accordingly. I was strong enough; I needed more muscular endurance.

It's worth noting that the contents of this book, as it relates to physiological and mental changes from strength training, apply to both men and women more or less equally. Yet bone loss has disproportionately adverse effects on women than men – being both more common and more severe – meaning women have a greater risk of developing osteoporosis. In fact, 33% of women are likely to experience an osteoporotic-related fracture in their lifetime, compared to only 20% of men.[31] This is largely because of the massive drop in levels of oestrogen in the blood post-menopause. This is nothing to be sniffed at, as oestrogen is the hormone that regulates the cells that break down old bone tissue and replace it with new.[32] With this understanding, the idea of taking it easy as you age is counterintuitive in some respects. While ridding yourself of unnecessary stressors is beneficial, so is a lifelong practice of active strength training to build bone mass and improve health. In general, bone loss is something women will want to pay particularly close attention to when thinking about the other ingredients that go into their training regime and lifestyle choices.

A study published in 2022 showed that people with osteoporosis were at an increased risk of contracting life-threatening illnesses and infections such as sepsis and pneumonia.[33] This shows how a wilful ignorance of how to engage in strength training safely and consistently can potentially lead to horrible circumstances. You could be forgiven for thinking you have plenty of time before this becomes a concern. Sadly not. Decline in bone mass starts from as early as thirty, so there's no time to waste.[34]

Summary

Scientific principles relating to how your body changes when training for strength and muscle growth are an essential consideration when designing a training plan suited to your needs. The fuel behind a sustainable programme is heavily reliant on lifestyle measures, the most important of which are good nutrition, adequate sleep and hydration.

SIX
The Risk Of Falling Off

In this chapter, you will learn more about why consistency is essential on your journey to transformation. You will also discover what goes into building consistency and the compound effects it has, which can be positive or negative depending on where your consistency manifests.

Don't abandon your plan

One of the most difficult things to do in the pursuit of a goal is to remain relentlessly consistent. I get it. It's hard work, with persistent sacrifice and, frankly, it's not always fun. When you start to think like this, in difficult moments, it's vital that you keep focused on the main goal because once you've achieved what you've set out to, the struggles of yesterday will become a hazy memory, disappearing in your rear-view mirror as you look down the road that opens up before you. Sure, there will be times where you have to take a hiatus from your programme for whatever reason – a restorative or ad hoc break is often a good thing – but what you can't do is abandon the journey entirely.

Remind yourself that the hard work and sacrifice is building you up, not breaking you down. This is a journey you embark on purposefully, not on a flippant impulse. You know the benefits, which is why you're doing it, so your feelings should follow your will – not the other way around. You will already have thousands of examples of where you have demonstrated this principle in your life. Take your morning rituals. It doesn't matter how you feel when you wake up, whether you're on top of the world or the world is on top of you, you still go into your bathroom and clean your teeth every morning. (At least, I hope you do.)

There are many ways you could rationalise falling off once you've started, but doing so will only show that your objectives were not as important to you as you believed and might need re-evaluating. Some people cite boredom as the reason for abandoning their training plans, perhaps thinking that attending the gym with friends is a sufficient reason to commit to the programme set before them. This is both a mistake and a misunderstanding of the psychological application required for difficult tasks.

Social factors are not a compelling enough reason to keep doing what you need to do to be in the weight room. They can certainly get you started, but that's about it, unless you seek out additional tools and knowledge. There are more suitable places for sociable activities and for people to congregate, where hard work isn't required.

If used appropriately, social collaboration will amplify your efforts and encourage you to keep your focus, but this depends on you knowing why you are strength training in the first place. The order here is key – motivation must come from within before it is reinforced by others, without it you'll confuse your means and ends.

So how do you remain as stimulated and committed as possible when it comes to your strength-training programme? I've found that there are predominantly two things that determine someone's continued efforts in a particular discipline or endeavour: problem-solving and desire, both of which are exemplified in Temi's story.

FOUR UNINTERRUPTED YEARS

Someone who has personified the subtle, yet impactful, effects of strength training is Temi Akomolafe. Our paths first crossed at university, where she started her journey, and I caught up with her recently to see how she's getting on, and her growth is admirable.

For the last four years, Temi has been training consistently four to six times a week – but she didn't start out that way. During university, Temi decided to start training (as most do) for aesthetic reasons, which were not a strong enough motivator to keep her consistently committed to her journey. Eventually, instead of trying to emulate the physical profiles she admired in other women, she settled in her mind that it was better to imitate the hard work and discipline they cultivated to get there. This meant she could switch her focus to something more pragmatic: routine – that's where the magic happened.

By her own admission, Temi knew that her natural tendency was to be lazy, stay comfortable and take the path of least resistance whenever the opportunity presented itself. She also knew that this wouldn't get her anywhere she would find satisfying. Instead, she sowed the seed by sticking to a challenging routine, and over the years, this blossomed into an unrelenting determination.

At work, this determination gave Temi the impetus to leave her unfulfilling job and seek a new challenge elsewhere. Once she'd found her new role, having the least experience and venturing beyond her comfort zone didn't inhibit her from putting herself forward for the most daunting tasks that nobody else in the team wanted to do. Within just one year, she was the regular recipient of praise and given high-profile responsibilities, thanks to the outstanding performance, reliability and value she brought to the team.

Trying new exercises in the gym, logging programme achievements and course correcting when her form or approach were wrong, allowed Temi to inadvertently use the gym as a training ground to shift her mindset to one of excellence in her approach towards all areas of her life. To ensure that she keeps her mind and body performing optimally, she applies the same level of rigour in prioritising her sleep, nutrition and heart health. Reflecting on her journey today, she remarks, 'I don't think I've realised how much that mindset has infiltrated my life. I don't believe I can't at least try to challenge myself in anything.'

Problem-solving and desire

When you are able to solve problems for yourself and others, you're viewed as a productive and valuable member of society. This is because we intuitively link value to solutions; if you are the one providing those solutions, it improves your self-perception and helps you to stay stimulated at the task you're involved. This applies to different people to varying degrees, but the general principle stands.

For example, at your job you may be the subject matter expert in an area that commands respect from your colleagues. They talk to you with respect and listen to what you have to say. They bring difficult problems to you because if anyone can solve them, it's you. Being able to solve problems and so being valued by others reinforces the value you place on yourself in your own mind and keeps you stimulated and motivated to work through challenges.

Let's say this isn't the case for you. Maybe your work is straightforward, perhaps even mundane. You don't have the opportunity to become an expert in your organisation or role, so you don't solve problems at work, but you continue anyway. Why? You continue because you get paid and that money helps you to solve other problems outside of your job and to continue to fund a full and active life – unemployment has consistently been found to negatively impact mental, physical and social health outcomes.[35] The problems you solve, or rather avoid, by working keep you stimulated to continue.

The equation is much simpler for desire. When you enjoy something, you are happy to do it and will do it consistently with vigour. When the thing being enjoyed is something productive, such as artistry, sports, fashion, vlogging or writing, you will notice that elements of problem-solving creep into your work and help you to advance your craft.

How does this apply to strength training? If you cast your mind back to Chapter Four, we noted the problems you're currently facing to which you're a direct contributor and how your strength training, when properly applied, can enhance your self-regulation and intangible results to stop you from being a barrier to achieving your goals – effectively, helping you to solve those problems. Throughout the book, I've highlighted the mental and physiological benefits of strength training. All these real changes breed real results; seeing positive results is hugely encouraging and makes your strength training a desirable activity, stimulating you in the deepest way possible.

THE CONTRAST BETWEEN TWO FRIENDS

The difference in outcomes between those who know why they are strength training and those with no substantive idea could not be illustrated more clearly than by two friends of mine.

On the one hand, there's Oscar. He is a large and overweight man; he's been that way since his youth and never had the desire to strength train. He didn't see it as enjoyable and certainly not as something relevant beyond a 'good' activity he needed to do to be healthy. The irony is, Oscar had many issues he wanted to resolve. He was insecure because of his weight and had found it difficult to focus and apply himself to the educational route he had chosen to pursue. He also wanted to be more productive than anyone else in our circle and be known as a guy who leads from the front. This was evident in the announcements he made in good faith about projects he was starting, only to later abandon them when the going got tough.

He would overcompensate for his insecurity through his social ambitions and sought validation from others. This has followed him, to a large extent, into adulthood.

At thirty, he is still at home with his parents when he would rather be living independently as he prepares himself for the next stage of his life. His career isn't anything he feels proud of and, frankly, he knows the lack of progress is his own fault.

But in his mind, he doesn't know what he could have done differently apart from work harder in school. Even after I've explained strength training to him in-depth, he still can't square that circle.

Then there's Andre. He was just as insecure and unfocused as Oscar was in school, but the difference was that Andre was underweight and much weaker than Oscar.

Andre had his own problems that he wanted to resolve, around his insecurity and anger issues. He would frequently flip out at his family members when they clashed and then later regret his inability to control his emotions.

Andre decided to pick up strength training as a healthy outlet for his boiling anger and put all the necessary tools and accountability measures in place so that he would remain consistent in solving this problem. He found that weightlifting would calm him down and the gym become a haven from all that was troubling him outside it. Andre became stronger and more self-aware, observing the changes in his body and mind.

Now when he became angry, he took a different approach. He wouldn't lash out like a wild animal. Instead, he would respond in a controlled and respectful way, where he could, and simply remove himself from the situation when he felt unable to stay and behave appropriately.

He told me that most of this came from him being able to see himself in the third person. 'I'm twice their size, how would it look if I started to assert my will over them and become domineering?'

His strength seemed to make him gentler, not more aggressive. But something even more profound happened, as he took away more than he intended to from strength training, and the character he'd forged in those early years followed him into adulthood.

Andre moved out of his parents' home at twenty-three, completed multiple degrees and professional qualifications and was earning £300,000 a year at twenty-seven. Every so often, he tells me that picking up those weights for the first time was one of the best things he ever did.

Need drives productivity

Before you read any further, take a moment to write a list of the things you think you need to live, generally. How many things on your list do you already have? The idea is that whatever it is you think you need, this is what will inspire you to put in maximal effort to get it. We human beings have much better success at working to achieve that which we believe we can't do without than that which we believe would be merely desirable. In essence, your perceived needs are what determine and drive your productivity.

Idleness hurts you

Let's say you understand all the physical, mental and social benefits of strength training and how it has the potential to radically change your trajectory. But even with this knowledge and the desire to follow through, you still find it difficult to remain consistent. You have good runs for a while and then stop training for equally as long, if not longer. You welcome gains to your body and mind, and then wave them goodbye once you become idle.

Why is this? You need to be honest with yourself. Barring exceptional circumstances, the reason why you start today and stop tomorrow is because you're being lazy. That kind of attitude will not serve you during this transformative phase. You must turn up to every session ready to work and your attendance needs to be regular and unbroken. Nobody likes to be told they're lazy; we don't even like to tell ourselves we're lazy. Instead, we say things like 'I can't be bothered', because it sounds softer, but it isn't helpful. If we only did the things we were *bothered* to do, we wouldn't get much done. The next time you want to say 'I can't be bothered', replace those words with 'I am lazy' – because that is what you're being. Let that truth wake you up and kick you into action. Lazy people don't achieve much – you have already proven to yourself that you know how to sweat.

A personal gauge of effort is a helpful tool on your strength-training journey. There is a yardstick that you take with you everywhere, which you can use to measure your training consistency. I recommend you pay close attention to it. The first time you picked up a heavy weight, you would have felt some discomfort in your hands; they may have even hurt a little. This mild injury to the cells on the outer layer of skin on your palms will have caused it to undergo a process called hyperkeratosis, a fancy word for 'thickening'. The more occurrences of mild injury and weight applied to these cells, the thicker the skin becomes. This is called a callus.[36]

Calluses develop to protect the underlying tissue in your hands. It wouldn't make sense to try and rid yourself of them if your training is of the type that produces them. Investing in a pair of protective gloves would be a better alternative. Some people don't like calluses. When I first started developing them as a teenager, I thought something was wrong with my hands, but now I've grown to love them. Every day I catch myself subconsciously running my thumbs across my calluses – they remind me that I'm on track. They are physiological trophies that I only get to keep if I continue training – if I stop, they start to disappear.

Another purpose they serve is as a tangible representation of the mental toughness I've formed as a result of enduring the discomfort of strength training. In that respect, the current state of the calluses on your hands reflects the conditioning of your mind. Use them as your laziness gauge. If they start disappearing, this could be the first sign that your strength of mind will soon follow suit.

The inevitable wall

There will come a point when you feel as though you are stagnating – your strength gains are slowing down and it's requiring more effort to maintain your current training regime. There is nothing to worry about.

If you're doing everything we've discussed and so are training to a decent standard, you will have already experienced some immense physical and psychological changes. But you're still a human being; there will be a point where you'll have reached your limits, and at some point, a decline will begin.

Sarcopenia is defined as an age-related involuntary loss of lean muscle mass, strength and function. There isn't a person on earth who won't be affected by it; it generally starts from the age of thirty.[37] Before you get too concerned, you should know that this happens at a pretty slow rate for the first couple of decades, where muscle mass decline is approximately 3–8% per decade.

This is where your judgement plays a key role, as no training programme can account for this without that level of awareness from you. If you start to feel as though you are overexerting yourself in the gym while maintaining your best practices, it could be time to start adjusting your training regime downward.

Strength training is a lifestyle, a form of exercise with great potential for longevity – you don't want to jeopardise that by pushing your body beyond its capabilities.

The good news is that the invisible characteristics you've developed up until now have come from your determined attempts and efforts to improve yourself through strength training. It doesn't matter how much weight you've logged in each workout. The important thing, no matter how strong you are, is that you continue to apply and benefit from the virtues born out of your training.

This is where all the information and data you've gathered will enable you to make an accurate assessment of your capabilities and the best way to push through the inevitable wall. Here, you're primarily concerned with the following:

- General science about the body's response to strength training
- Assessment of your body's response to strength training
- Any medical or health issues you may be dealing with
- Lifestyle factors such as hydration, diet, sleep and recovery time

As I've already mentioned, consistency is the backbone of accurate and quality training data, but both need careful attention and care if you are going to become more informed about how strength training positively impacts your physical and mental health.

Physical rewards

Progressive overload is a core pillar of your training and one that can only come through consistent efforts. Only when your muscles have adapted to the stimulus they experience on a regular basis, will they be ready to handle more weight. If you take consistency out of the equation, progressive overload becomes impossible and your prospective achievements get further and further away.

When it comes to the gym, an effective way to keep yourself accountable is to diarise your workouts for the week in your calendar. From a psychological perspective, this is more effective than keeping a vague to-do list because a calendar accounts for time and forces you to limit your choices and work within the confines of each twenty-four-hour period so that you get the important things done.

Research undertaken by a productivity company found that 41% of items on to-do lists are never completed.[38] You can't be only turning up to your workouts 41% of the time. That would make progressive overload incredibly difficult and hurt your chances of becoming stronger. We know that muscle is body armour and studies have found that strength-training programmes can reduce your risk of injury by 33% so make sure to diarise your workouts and watch as your adherence to your training schedule vastly improves.[39]

TOO MUCH TO BEAR

When I was younger, I had some recurring issues with inconsistency. I decided to implement some practical measures to refocus my priorities on my training.

The main addition was making sure that I'd noted in my personal calendar what days and times I would train the following week. I'd then highlight these entries in a specific colour to differentiate my workout programme from the other demands on my time.

I had this meticulous way of making sure that I only scheduled that which I intended to do, and once it was written down with a time to be completed, I considered myself bound to make good on my word.

It was one of those honourable virtues we talked about earlier that flowed into other areas of my life, and it taught me to think long and hard about a decision before I committed to it.

I used this diary method to see just how strong I could get on the weighted pull-up. After I went out and bought the strongest weighted belt I could find, I started doing pull-ups with a 20kg plate hanging from my waist.

That soon got easy, so I added another 5kg plate and continued to push myself. It felt good. My grip strength was getting much tighter and my back was getting thicker.

I believed there was still more room to grow, so I continued to overload the weight hanging from my waist until I needed liquid chalk to help increase the friction between my hands and the bar I would hang on.

Within a year, I had reached what I felt was my limit. After a brief warm-up to begin my workout sessions, I'd walk over to the iron plates and make two trips back to where I would do my weighted pull-ups. On the first trip, I'd bring back two 20kg plates in each hand; then, on the second trip, I'd have another 20kg plate in one hand and a 15kg plate in the other. I was performing three sets of five reps that were excellent form, wide-gripped pull-ups, with an additional 75kg hanging from my waist. I weighed 97kg at the time and would often have people ask me how I'd got so strong. After giving them the same techniques I've outlined in this book, they started to see impressive results of their own.

A word of caution, though: be careful. I had no idea the effect the added weight was having on the chain attached to my belt. One day when I got ready to perform my usual weighted pull-ups with the 75kg attachment, I was three reps into the second set when the chain gave out and all the weights crashed down to the floor. Every head swivelled in my direction. 'What was that?' I heard someone exclaim. I came down, unharmed, to find the gym owner walking over.

'You alright?' he asked. 'Yeah, don't worry. I'm OK, thank you,' I replied, thinking he was coming to check on me. He was actually more concerned about his damaged floor.

Summary

It's now clear that you are only going to obtain the quality of the data you need to inform your training in a way that will work efficiently for you. Remembering your needs and the personal problems you're solving will help keep you motivated on the difficult days. Without this, negligence is likely, progress starts to wane and frustration sets in when you realise that you may need to rebuild. At some point you'll hit the wall, and this is the perfect time to regroup and adjust accordingly. If you persist through these challenges, you'll be able to experience more of the physical benefits provided by strength training.

SEVEN

If It's Not Documented, It's Not Done

In this chapter, you will learn why workout records are so valuable and why artificial intelligence is the best way to keep these. Let's be real, most people don't keep any records of their workouts let alone detailed records. In fact, some estimate that at least 95% of people don't keep any records of their workouts whatsoever.[40] If you fall into that camp of non-recorders, I understand. On the one hand, before now you may have struggled to grasp the significance of keeping an accurate journal and what exactly that does for you. On the other hand, keeping a detailed log of your workout activities is tiresome, boring and more admin than you probably signed up for when you joined the gym.

If there are two things that will guarantee you won't do something, they are:

1. Not being convinced of its value

2. A difficult path to completing what should be an easy task

In light of the above, what you really need to know is why logging your workouts is beneficial for you, beyond having a pile of documents, which we will find out shortly; then, you want to find the easiest possible way to do what is required to reap the rewards that you know are on the other side of this action.

The value of workout records

There are three main reasons why workout records are valuable:

1. They keep you motivated.

2. They advise next actions.

3. They help you identify patterns.

Motivation

Tracking your progress towards your goals is just as important as setting them in the first place – arguably even more so, because if you set goals without checking on how close you're getting to them, you're likely to fail to achieve them or give up altogether.

By contrast, if you're religiously monitoring your progress with less focus on a set end point, without knowing for sure how far you're trying to go, you end up developing a mindset of pushing yourself further each day because wherever that end point is, it's always just out of reach. I've seen this play out in some of my most successful friends, who have ended up achieving more than they initially set out to.

What we want is both the end goal and the information about our progress in getting there – both are valuable. Looking back over a visual reminder of what you have achieved doesn't just make you feel good, it also encourages you to keep going.

Next actions

As sharp as your mind may be, it is no match for the bluntest pencil. Let's face it, we overestimate how good our memories are all the time, yet forgetting things does not help us to make changes to our methods.

Think about how frustrated you'd feel if you asked someone to recall something important only for them to come back with, 'I can't remember.' Having workout data will give you an easy to access reference point that can advise you on what alterations to make to your training, when to make them and how to go about it safely and effectively. It will also let you know when you're stagnating, which can happen for different reasons – the data enables you to investigate. If there is reason to slow down and avoid injury risk, then you'll have a solid empirical basis on which to make that decision. You won't be able to judge this accurately without records. If you've met your targets and not injured yourself up until now, then consider yourself lucky – but remember that luck is not sustainable and you may need these records in the future.

Patterns

There are two ways to identify patterns, and keeping a record of information about your workouts as well as your lifestyle will help you do both. The first way is to see how your strength training is affected by other lifestyle factors such as sleep, diet, work and relationships. The second way is simply the reverse: reviewing your strength training and identifying how it is affecting other areas of your life. This will help you dial into, and possibly scale back on, factors that are unique to your life and circumstances.

We're all affected by different things in different ways, which is why a tailored approach is always the most sensible. For example, an argument at work may cause you to be anxious and restless, so you have a poor night's sleep before your workout. If you go ahead with the workout as planned, your training log may show that you struggled to keep up; with some careful consideration of your training history, you can deduce why. There are many possible scenarios you could experience and only be able to make sense of through having an accurate record of your training efforts and outcomes.

The role of artificial intelligence in training data

Admittedly, there are some limitations to recording your workouts yourself, which are obvious when you think about it. First, there is the issue of precise observation. For example, at the most basic level, you don't exactly know how your form differs from one repetition to the next, and where the variation is too large to be considered a successful repetition. For the odd repetition this is not too much of a concern, but multiply it across dozens of workouts and you have a problem – especially when you consider that improper form is one of the core reasons for injuries sustained from strength training.[41]

Second, there is the issue of limited observation. What do I mean by that? There is only so much information you can gather through merely observing an exercise. The more important information, which provides far greater utility, is the kind that can only be picked up by sophisticated technology and artificial intelligence (AI). For example, if your left quad looks slightly bigger than your right, and you wanted to see what the weight distribution between both legs was while you're performing your squats, that will require technology. This type of technology is also able to provide insights and recommendations to help you re-position yourself for a balanced, safer and more stable performance.

AI is easily the most exciting innovation of the last few years, and it's only just getting started. People are beginning to grasp the astounding capabilities and potential of this technology, which can completely redesign our usual way of doing things, saving us time and money, flagging hidden risks and providing more accurate information on which to base decisions, to name a few.

AI is not just the future – it's now. Virtually every industry is incorporating some aspect of AI into their processes, but it looks like strength training is late to the party. I can understand why. Trying to innovate is no small feat in an environment where you are capturing and delivering accurate data to many individuals in a confined space while freely moving objects are being thrown around by multiple people. It's a huge challenge, but it's not impossible.

Throughout the book we've addressed the first reservation outlined at the beginning of this chapter regarding why you may choose not to bother with workout data. The second reservation, that it's too difficult, essentially disappears with the advent of the nascent and mass-produced technology – specifically, machine learning, deep learning and artificial neural networks. Don't worry, you don't need to know exactly what they are and how they work, but you should know how they can impact, in a practical way, your strength training.

On the backend, your training facility would have some technology installed that is designed to establish communication paths between you and the equipment you're using. Most people have their mobile phones or smartwatches with them while training – you'll need one of those, for two reasons:

1. To see all your strength training performance insights in real-time through the app; it receives this data from the facility's backend technology.

2. To act as the final component that identifies you as the person training, without you having to do anything.

Once equipped with your phone or smartwatch, the rest is simple. Train as usual and watch the information you've never before had access to roll through your app's data feed, capturing and downloading it all for your current and future use. It sounds like magic, and in a way it is. This level of insight can transform the way you think and approach holistic health and wellness. Even without digitalisation, the value of awareness around your physical activity is pivotal.

LESSONS FROM THE DIARY

A friend of mine, James, was a half-hearted gym-goer, but because he was so genetically blessed, he didn't need to do much work to appear more in shape than the average Joe. The issue with James was that he wouldn't always feel the same when he was doing his workouts, which led him to acquire an enduring irregularity. Some days he would feel so full of energy that his scheduled workout programme for the day seemed like merely a warm-up. On other days, he would feel so lethargic that he'd literally be dragging his heels to the gym – if he went at all. As you can imagine, he didn't perform well on those occasions. His form was sloppy and his attention was elsewhere. This affected his mind–muscle connection and, on more than a few occasions, led to unusual spasms in the muscle group he was training.

Despite this, James wanted to become stronger than he had ever been. He wasn't particularly interested in becoming the most chiselled guy on the block, but he did want to be strong so he could be relied on to be physically helpful to others who needed it.

One day, when James was struggling to get through his workout, I asked him why he never seemed to take stock of his workout or the things which were potentially affecting it.

'Too much effort, and besides it probably won't help much,' he replied.

Without missing a beat, I said, 'Don't you think it would help you find the reasons for your wild fluctuations in energy? Look at where your feet are placed when you're holding that bar, you're going to hurt yourself and put your back out. Then you won't be strong anymore.'

His internal musings were written all over his face and shortly after he started documenting his workouts and lifestyle. It took him two weeks to realise that the reason he felt so sluggish on those off days was because he would eat a large and spicy dinner less than three hours before he went to sleep. This meant he would wake up with horrible sleep inertia and take the residual effects to the gym in the morning.

Once he made some minor but impactful changes to his diet and mealtimes, his rejuvenated energy levels meant he couldn't keep out of the gym. He was stronger and more disciplined than ever.

Different pieces, same puzzle

In the supplementation of AI, you need to be diligent enough to take note of the seemingly trite occurrences of life, especially in the application that houses your data. These don't occur in a vacuum, only affecting you in a one-dimensional way. If that were the case, it would be much easier to figure out cause and effect. But it isn't.

A beautiful sunset can trigger nostalgic memories, bringing to mind old friends of whom you were fond, providing an opening to reach out and re-connect.

This is just one example of a seemingly insignificant moment having a profound effect. I'm not suggesting that you start analysing every experience you have and recording it in your training database, but you should be all over your routine so that you know precisely where your gold dust is. This kind of knowledge is empowering in helping you sail smoothly towards success while at the same time eliminating the obstacles that would impede your progression.

There is something unique about the role that strength training plays in this. It is training you do to your body in a facility to reap results outside of it. The strength you gain is something you carry with you everywhere you go. Central to your training is your overall health. This is the starting point – by caring about your health, you are more likely to care about your home, your relationships and your environment.

Once you have some valuable data related specifically to *your* life and performance, you will naturally start to engage in problem-solving without thinking too hard about it. By simply taking time to articulate what your pain points are, you have had to take time to understand the issues you may be facing and how you contribute to their continued existence. These will be fresh in your mind as you find yourself wrestling with how you can take what you have learned about yourself from your training and use the positive attributes you have demonstrated that you possess, and use it to change any circumstances you are unhappy with.

Your personality framework

There are five distinct personality traits that psychologists use to assess our behaviour depending on the degrees to which we exhibit each trait. These are:

- Extraversion – how sociable you are
- Conscientiousness – how diligent, organised and productive you are
- Agreeableness – how empathetic and compassionate you are
- Openness – how receptive you are to new ideas
- Neuroticism – how anxious or depressed you are

Research has found that 78% of the 6,800 adult samples wanted to increase their levels of the first four traits and decrease their level of neuroticism.[42] This makes sense, as people tend to be happier and healthier when they are not anxious or depressed.[43]

In the past, psychologists believed that personality was largely fixed and couldn't be changed, but that belief is no longer the prevailing one. Brent Roberts, a leading expert on personality change, explained that the deep-seated desire on the part of many people to think personality is unchanging is because it simplifies your world in a way that is quite nice because it allows you to abdicate your responsibility for certain behaviours.[44] We now have evidence that suggests your personality traits can be moved in a more positive direction, if desired, by adopting certain behaviours.[45]

What does this mean for you and why is it relevant to your strength training? Let's return again for a moment to the pain points you noted to which you are a contributor. These will have been determined by your personality, so to make changes you might want to consider where you sit on any, some or all those five dimensions and if there's anything you're not happy with.

Fortunately, you already have a set of keys to unlock the door to this change – your strength training programme. For me and many others, strength training has been a pivotal force for positive change in our lives.

If we assume for a moment that you wish to make improvements in all five personality dimensions, then there are ways in which you can do this through your training. Yet it's only *intentional* work done with a degree of self-awareness that will yield the best results. Let's look at how strength training can help us incorporate behaviours that can lead to small but powerful changes to our personality, taking each dimension in turn.

Extraversion

People who are highly extraverted like to start conversations and feel energised when other people are around. To be clear, there is nothing wrong with introversion, or being an introvert generally, but certainly there are situations and times in life where being able to easily talk to and engage with others is necessary and/or beneficial. The gym couldn't be an easier place to start a conversation. I'm always having them. It is easier to start a conversation than you might think, and I would suggest that one of the reasons you don't want to train alone at home (if you could) is because you don't get the same buzz as you do from being around other people also working towards their goals.

Conscientiousness

People who are highly conscientious are often those who pay close attention to details and enjoy having a set schedule to follow.[46]

Keeping a detailed workout journal will force you to be more attentive to details so that you can make the necessary adjustments for your own benefit. This goes hand in hand with having – and sticking to – a schedule, so that you can have more consistent and reliable data, with accurate and actionable details.

Agreeableness

People who are very agreeable will assist others in need of help and enjoy contributing to the happiness of people around them.

How many times have you had the opportunity to help your fellow gym-goers, and how many times have you been helped by someone in return? If you ever see me in your gym, I may need some liquid chalk from you – I'm always forgetting mine.

Openness

People who are very open will often be willing to try new things and be focused on tackling new challenges.

This is precisely why you are in the gym lifting weights in the first place. Strength training is a challenge, one that often leads to you trying new things in order to better your results, accommodate your lifestyle choices and avoid injuries.

Neuroticism

People who score low for neuroticism tend to appear more relaxed, deal well with stress and are seen as emotionally stable.

We have already looked at data that shows strength training is a formidable equaliser for stress, depression and anxiety for many people in situations and circumstances that make it a sensible and appropriate activity to introduce. Unsurprisingly, this is also typically one of the main reasons why people commit themselves fully to the process.

Having said all of this, the objective isn't to permanently swing yourself to the other end of the spectrum for each personality dimension, but rather by balancing between any extremes you've identified in yourself, or even by simply adjusting your personality depending on the situation you're presented with. This doesn't happen overnight; it takes careful practice and you might find it encouraging to know that these changes do not need to be large to be transformative.

FAILING TO SUCCEED

I had a difficult time during my early days of studying to qualify as an accountant. At twenty-three, I had packed up my dearest belongings and set up shop on a neighbouring island where I hoped to become a bona fide member of a global accounting body.

The trouble was, I hated numbers and vowed to myself that after my compulsory education I wouldn't go into a profession that required me to do much computation because it was boring. Yet there I was, enrolled on an accountancy training contract, and I couldn't go back home without that qualification.

The first exam didn't involve any numbers and it was easy enough for everyone to pass comfortably. I passed with the highest mark in my cohort; it was a great feeling, but it quickly evaporated to be replaced with despair when the next exam, on financial accounting, did involve numbers. I wasn't doing so well in those classes and as exam day drew closer, I had this ominous feeling that I wouldn't like the result once it was done. I was so stressed that I stopped going to the gym altogether to 'focus'. I was clearly confused about what purpose weight training was serving in my life at that point.

When it came time to finally sit the exam, I failed. I went from cheesing like I'd won a small fortune to frantically dealing with the admin of scheduling a retake. The policy of the firm I was working for was that after three fails, you were fired.

My confidence had taken a serious beating, which affected my ability to study for the retake, and on top of that I knew if I failed again I would be one failed exam away from losing my job and having to fly back home with my tail between my legs. Distressed, I worried about how I would manage the more difficult exams that lay ahead when I was already struggling this early on. I realised that I had to start going to the gym again to blow off this steam. I didn't even recognise myself anymore. Anyone who knows me would describe me as a calm and collected, easy-going kind of guy, so who was this? Behind closed doors, I was a panicked mess.

Once I restarted my training, I found that I was able to manage the stress in a healthy way, which gave me a clearer mind when it was time to study. It was still shaky at times, but it was a vast improvement. Exam day came again and, although I was anxious, I knew the only way around this obstacle was to pass, so I gave it my best shot. All I remember seeing on my results sheet was the word 'pass'. Relief doesn't even begin to describe what I felt in that moment. I had lived to fight another day, no searching for plane tickets just yet. I'd also cracked my code: strength training was an instrument for my success, so I needed to use it accordingly.

I passed the eleven remaining (and more difficult) exams without a single fail.

Summary

You now know that workout records are valuable because they keep you motivated, advise next actions and help you identify patterns. Even in the strength training arena, AI is fast becoming the mode used to save time and deliver huge quantities of valuable information. However, this is not a substitute for paying attention to your qualitative experiences and how they affect your workout approach on any given day. Doing these things will furnish you with the information you need to use your gym and strength training as an incubator to make slight but favourable personality adjustments.

PART THREE
THE REBIRTH

EIGHT
New Kinds Of Challenges

In this chapter, you will learn how the strategies we've talked about, using the various kinds of data we have looked at, all culminate in and contribute to a stronger resolve when facing challenges outside of the gym.

The sooner you pick up and explore the things taught in this book, the further you'll be able to go. You may even encourage the younger generation coming behind you to adopt and cultivate these same healthy habits. Life is challenging by nature and I'm constantly amazed at how naturally resilient we humans are. You wonder how some people are able to wake up and face another day when you hear of their struggles; strangely, many are doing this incidentally, with no sure or proven way to strengthen their resolve. They're just doing it.

The difference that gathering actionable knowledge makes to not only being able to endure certain challenges but to thrive on them, is truly exhilarating. Your mind is a precious thing; it's the ethereal centre of you, where you find solutions to your problems and determine which course of action you should take at any given moment.

Neuroscientific evidence tells us that a physically inactive lifestyle impacts negatively on brain health, while physical activity releases neurotransmitters and a molecule called brain-derived neurotrophic factor (BDNF), which increases new neurons, attention, memory and, critically for us, motivation.[47] There are numerous studies that show how, even in children, physical activity enhances brain activity. For example, research undertaken with children aged nine to eleven showed that four-minute physical activity intervals during class improved selective attention, a crucial factor in learning.[48] What's exciting is what effect this enhanced brain activity, coupled with the motivation it provides, can have on you, even from a young age.

MR PERFECT'S IMPERFECT PREDICTIONS

I was always a quiet and timid child and would often doubt my capabilities. In the final years of primary school, I was in awe of the smartest kids in the class who seemed to do well on every test, while I was just above average. We all sat in the same class learning the same thing and getting the same homework, so why were they outperforming everyone else so drastically?

This was a conundrum I couldn't solve. It could have been that they had extra tuition, more help with their homework, or they were just gifted and talented in academia. Whatever the case, I thought I may as well keep trying my best. In my final year of primary school, all the kids in my class were getting ready to take their 11+ exam – a selective test that a child had to pass if they (or their parents) wanted to attend a fee-paying or state grammar school the following academic year. The idea behind the tests was to identify the brightest students and provide them with a superior education. Whether this works is debatable, but nevertheless my mum wanted me to have the option to go.

This was a stressful time for any child of that age and, a few months before the big day, I remember the brightest kids in the class asking our teacher, Mr Perfect (his actual name!), whether he thought they would pass the exam. He reassured them that they would be fine. I plucked up the courage to ask him, 'What about me, sir? Do you think I'll pass?' I will never forget his response. He took a blank look at me, shook his head and said, 'No.' Ouch.

Around this time, an uncle of mine from Nigeria would occasionally come to visit us. When he did, we would do exercises together, which consisted of push-ups, squats and core work. Inadvertently, he unlocked a whole new world for me that would help me focus better and give me more confidence to embrace challenges.

Meanwhile, my mum enrolled me in extra tuition to give me the best chance of success. It was a tough year, but exercising in the way I was taught by my uncle seemed to be helping my learning, though I still wasn't sure how I'd fare in the exam, Mr Perfect's words replaying in the back of my head.

Exam day came, and I had no idea how I'd done. When we finally got the results in the post, I got to the letter first so I could brace myself for disappointment before showing my mum.

'Dear Mr Ajanaku, I am delighted to offer you a place. . .'

I stopped reading. Euphoric and relieved, I skipped into the kitchen to show my mum. Her scream of excitement is still ringing in my ears.

Ironically, Mr Perfect had been wrong.

Goal realism

There is an often-cited maxim that you can do anything you put your mind to. While this will undoubtedly drive many successes, you will inherently know that it isn't true. There are some things that you'll find are just physically and / or logistically impossible. Then there are things where, once you've assessed their feasibility, you conclude are highly unlikely and not worth the effort.

This doesn't need to be disheartening, because when you look at the things you desperately want to achieve, you'll probably find that they are not only possible, but they are also within reaching distance.

We don't tend to put things that we know aren't practicable high on our list of desires. We instead focus our efforts in areas where we know we are likely to get the biggest payoffs; these will be different for everyone and depend on the unique variables that you bring to the table. For example, I may be a keen enthusiast of hyper-photorealism and be extremely well versed in deciphering the emotional intent the artist is trying to convey through their masterpiece. On the other hand, if I do not have the dexterity that comes from stellar hand-eye coordination coupled with a detailed vision, it would be a waste of time for me to try and become one of the world's most prolific hyper-photorealistic artists, though I can still appreciate the artistry.

Aiming for goals that are within the realm of your capabilities is the surest way to be confident that you will eventually hit them. It's not for anyone else to tell you what you are and are not capable of; this will be a product of your motivation, skills, time commitment and resources.

Self-doubt and your biggest driver

The chances are that you have experienced self-doubt at one point or another, perhaps when faced with a task, project or event in which you were expected to perform well. You may have questioned whether you were worthy of success or if you even had it in you to bring about the result you were seeking or the performance that was expected. This is a normal phenomenon that happens to all of us; we are not superheroes and we don't need to be.

Self-doubt in and of itself is related to a more general perception of yourself and your abilities, which is sometimes not founded on anything substantive. When you're trying to do something specific, this can manifest as a fear of failure. This is not an aimless and abstract emotion but rather one directed towards or attached to a particular effort, event or task.

Providing your fear of failure is not crippling, there are several research studies that support the notion that it can be a valuable contributor to human behaviour and, specifically, that it stimulates people to adopt certain types of behaviour that predispose them to success.[49] This is good news for us, my friend. From the perspective of your pursuits that have no direct relation to your physical efforts, strength training is a behaviour that can seem immaterial at best. But strength training is multifaceted. It has been the subject of much study, which has evidenced benefits in managing pain, improving cognitive ability, mitigating anxiety and depression, lowering the risk of heart and circulatory issues, preventing injury, enhancing posture and balance and bettering sleep quality, to name just a few. When self-doubt and fear of failure are harnessed in a healthy way, challenges take on a whole new meaning.

THE STRESS MANAGEMENT
OF A BUSINESS OWNER

A close friend of mine, Ellie, understands the relevance of strength training better than most. She came from a challenging background, growing up in a two-bed house on a council estate with eleven family members. If that wasn't challenging enough, they lived in a dangerous part of the city and many family members were involved in crime. This exposed Ellie to danger, heartbreak and ultimately inescapable problems that affected her livelihood.

What Ellie lacked in education, she made up for in raw determination and ambition. She wanted out, but not just for herself – she wanted to take as many of her family members with her as possible and provide them with an education-focused solution that would sustain their livelihoods. A tall order, right?

She got to work building her own company specialising in EdTech and has long moved away from the area she grew up in. She moved into an office in a top financial district and practically lives there five days a week, sometimes not going home at all during the working week. Her office is also right next to her high-end gym, where she doesn't miss a single session.

One day, when we were eating lunch, I looked at her and said, 'Ellie, you're flat out but you've done so well. Why do you apply so much effort? What's driving you?'

She sighed deeply, as if the answer was a struggle just to think about. 'I'm scared,' she replied. 'I just don't want to fail. I know where I came from and I just can't go back there.'

I understood the sentiment all too well because it's fear of failure that drives me too. I can still recall the wonderful 'meeting of minds' moment we shared when I asked how she manages to keep performing so well when the stress appears to be mounting.

She explained, in a profound revelation, 'Health is the backbone of any success I've experienced until now and I feel healthy when I feel strong, which is why I'm always in the gym.' I knew that we were speaking the same language.

Aspirations

Unfortunately, there are plenty of unhelpful platitudes around that suggest a proposed course of action without any practical insight as to how this thing might be achieved. Think of, 'You miss 100% of the shots you don't take', or, 'Sacrifice today for a better tomorrow'. This kind of thinking doesn't get anyone anywhere. I'm sure you can point to at least half a dozen people you know who have said they are working on a project that they never seem to get around to, much less complete to a good standard. In most cases, this is down to a poor execution strategy.

A study conducted in 2020 found that 76% of participants who took time to write down their goals, created a plan of action and built a support system to hold themselves accountable, went on to successfully achieve those goals.[50] The premise of this book is about showing you how to use the vehicle of data and strength training to transcend your physical goals, so let's now look at how we can apply the principles we've discussed so far to some of your other aspirations.

When you first have the idea of wanting to achieve something, there's usually only a cloudy outline of what success looks like in your mind. It can't stay that way. This vision of what you think success looks like will have gaps and be ill-defined. You may feel certain of what you want to achieve today but when you're faced with new information and novel situations, your idea of success could change with it.

The word I love to use when describing being absolutely clear on my objectives is that I want to be perspicuous. The reason I love this word is because (i) it is underused and has the effect of conveying a deeper level of clarity and (ii) unless you know what the word means, it isn't clear in itself, which is a reminder to myself that I must be.

The way to be perspicuous in your aspirations is to write your vision down on paper or type it up on a computer. This forces you to organise your thoughts and articulate exactly what you want and how you plan to get there, which requires careful introspection and knowledge.

Just by doing this, you are 42% more likely to achieve your goals.[51] If attaining them will take you some time, this is the first exercise you must do to focus your efforts and avoid wasting time before you set out on the journey.

Equipping yourself

Just as there is no use in trying to engage in strength training with poor information and methods, there is no use in working towards your personal goals with the wrong resources or information. Misinformation and exploitative practices exist in every industry out there. This makes your life more difficult when it comes to trying to vet the people and resources that can potentially advance your progress towards your goals. This is why it's so important to equip yourself properly – identifying the right people, resources and information can save you hundreds, even thousands of hours of wasted time.

It is sad to see how many slick-talking, charismatic personas are able to successfully pedal falsehoods on the backs of those who unwittingly connect them to others who want what they've got. I'm not suggesting that no one is to be trusted, but I do propose that it would be wise to look objectively at the data and information available before coming to the most reasonable conclusion.

One of the cardinal rules I have developed, based on my experience and observations, and something that will significantly reduce your chances of ending up ill-equipped for achieving your goals, is to only spend time with and on credible people and resources. Don't underestimate the power of this rule's simplicity. We are generally not great critical thinkers and are often led by our emotions. This makes it all the more important that you question and test the efficacy of what you're hearing and seeing before investing more of your time and/or money. This is precisely why we adopt a strength-training approach that is rooted in scientific research and technology.

Persevering consistently

It's not difficult to start something, anything. Many well-intentioned people gather themselves in a burst of excitement to embark on a grand masterplan that they anticipate will bring them joy, fulfilment and status. What's more of a challenge is persevering with it after the initial excitement has died down. This is often short lived and all that's left are the dry bones of what was once a dream full of life. In most cases, the lack of methodology in place at the starting point of the journey had already doomed them to fail.

There are some instances where everything necessary for you to make a dream a reality seems to be in place and all that is left for you to do is execute it. Where that is the case and you find that it's still a challenge to persevere consistently, you first need to acknowledge that this is normal – it is the call to be relentless in your pursuit that filters out those who really want something from the pretenders.

A well-used tip is to regularly talk about what you're going to do with anyone who will listen, in the general course of your conversations. People always want to hear about what people are getting up to, but you're doing this for you – it's an accountability exercise. You will either elevate your esteem in others' eyes when you deliver on your word, or your reputation may be marred when you fail to honour what you said you would do. Giving yourself this kind of accountability is one of the most compelling ways to keep you on the right path.

If you are still unable to demonstrate consistency in your venture, then you need to think about whether this is something you actually want. There is no shame if you decide that it isn't, but you should find this out as soon as possible to avoid wasting any more of your time.

Documenting diligently

As you can see, there is a lot going on when it comes to setting your targets and doing what is required to achieve them. Add to that the fact that life is busy and we are rarely engaged in just one endeavour at once, and how do you have any idea if you're on track? It's impossible to know if and how far you have progressed if you aren't keeping accurate records to capture those all-important details. If you're using AI, you won't need to worry about being diligent in your documentation, as it will be taking care of this for you. You just need to refocus your efforts on turning up and putting in the effort.

I've found there are three main reasons for keeping hold of your workout logs and maintaining a history of training data, which are: for reference, accountability and encouragement.

First, the evidence documented can cover anything from things said to things done. Having this as a reference point gives you scope to adjust your approach and advance your position as you hit your milestones. It can be extremely valuable in helping to identify health risks during medical appraisals, providing practitioners with the exercise data they need to formulate their interventions. Keeping these records also supports transparency, as it keeps you accountable in the moments of questioning and monitoring.

The most attractive reason of all though, is having an audit trail of exactly where you've come from to where you currently are in pursuit of your goals. This provides an encouraging and perceptible reminder to you of your capabilities, casting a light on the growth process and allowing you to see it in a way that you inevitably miss while it's happening.

Summary

When goal setting for your physical measures, ensure you are leveraging your unique set of advantages. This will make it more likely that you will meet and exceed your goals. You may experience self-doubt, but this can be harnessed to act as a stimulus rather than an inhibitor. To help with this, you must be clear on what you are trying to achieve and aim to use objectively verifiable information where possible. It is easier to persevere when you have a substantive basis for action. By being able to review an audit of your progress and see where you have come from, it will be easier to forecast where you are going.

NINE
The Mind Sharpener

In this chapter, you will learn about some common themes related to mental resilience and how to apply a number of key principles to increase your ability to successfully tackle new challenges.

Defining mental toughness

Jim Loehr, one of the leading sports psychologists of the twentieth century, defined 'toughness' as the 'ability to consistently perform towards the upper range of your talent and skill regardless of competitive circumstances'.[52] This definition assumes not only that you need some degree of skill and talent to be mentally tough, but that you are also fully aware of the extent of your technical and physical capabilities. I tend to agree with this notion, and every time I'm confronted with a challenging situation I default to an assessment of whether I believe I am capable of coming out the other end triumphant.

Contrary to popular belief, mental toughness has nothing to do with being cold and emotionless, nor does it have anything to do with developing a killer instinct, so let's dispel those myths from the get-go. Navy SEALs are arguably the toughest men on the planet. They must endure unfathomable amounts of pain, meet the demands of challenges they have never before experienced and risk their lives every day – and that's just during BUD/S training that must be completed before one actually becomes a SEAL. In fact, between 2013 and 2016, more SEALs died in training than in combat.[53] There's no denying that this level of mental toughness is off the charts.

But most of us are not aspiring to be Navy SEALs. Does this mean that we don't have or even need mental toughness? Absolutely not. The degree to which your mental toughness is measured is relative to the objectives you are trying to achieve, this could be:

- Running a marathon

- Learning a new instrument

- Changing your dietary habits

- Starting a new venture

- Picking up a new language

- Writing your first book

Whatever it may be, once the picture of what you're trying to accomplish is clear in your mind and on paper, it will be easier for you to develop the mental toughness necessary to achieve your goals through action.

Emotions – the enemy of mental toughness

It couldn't be more obvious that emotions are a barrier to your development of mental toughness, and yet most people completely disregard this in their journey to fortifying their mind.

Typically, people decide at some point in their lives that they want to do something difficult because they like the idea of the rewards it will bring. It doesn't take long for the appeal of the challenge they've set themselves to start warring with how they feel at a given moment – tired, run down, demotivated, lazy or what have you. This would be an opportune time to stop, think and realise that we feel some kind of emotion 90% of the time, and these emotions are often changing.[54] Contrast a challenge with a task, which is emotionally neutral and doesn't change at all in its level of difficulty, and you quickly realise that your emotions are an awful thing to determine your behaviour.

The quicker you understand that your emotions can't be trusted to lead you to success, and start taking responsibility for your emotions by allowing them to follow your volition rather than the other way around, you will put yourself on an accelerated path to developing mental toughness. I've also squared this in my own mind and gained greater control over my feelings by using the analogy that being easily wound up or frustrated is like owning a TV and giving the remote to someone else. Putting this into practice doesn't mean that you will become entirely immune to the natural fluctuations in your emotional state, but it does mean that, with practice, your emotions become a lot less erratic, helping you to keep calm and stay the course.

In the UK, over eight million people are suffering from anxiety at any one time.[55] That's almost the whole population of London. Can you imagine walking around in a city like London knowing that every person whose eyes you meet is suffering from generalised anxiety disorder? To make matters worse, less than half of these people successfully access treatment,[56] for a whole host of reasons we can't get into. Anxiety typically manifests in feelings of worry, fear, nervousness, apprehension and foreboding. It's perfectly normal to experience feelings of anxiety when circumstances call for it, but prolonged symptoms may indicate a deeper issue.

Unfortunately, depression is a pervasive public health issue and even more people suffer from depression than anxiety in the UK.[57] The question is, does strength training help to combat anxiety and depression? Leaving aside subjective opinions and personal experiences, a meta-analysis of several studies meeting the criteria for quality research on this topic found a weight of available evidence supporting the conclusion that resistance training is a meaningful measure for reducing anxiety symptoms in healthy adults. These results are not dissimilar from those of the investigation that was done into the effects of resistance training on clinically depressed adults. In four of these studies, the results were unanimous in identifying large reductions of depressive symptoms, and there were another six trials that observed an improvement in self-esteem.[58] This isn't mere coincidence. There are inherent characteristics of strength training that have holistic benefits.

Finding comfort in discomfort

The reason many people love strength training is because it's a training ground for more than just strength. One of the best ways to understand your motivation to adopt certain behaviours is the framework of Self-Determination Theory (SDT). SDT proposes that the degree to which you experience motivation determines the place it occupies on the autonomous continuum, as illustrated below.

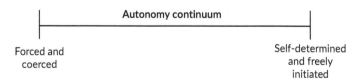

Autonomy continuum

Forced and coerced

Self-determined and freely initiated

145

Autonomy simply means how freely initiated the behaviour is. There are intrinsic and extrinsic components on this continuum. Intrinsic components are those which derive from the sheer pleasure and satisfaction of engaging in the behaviour itself,[59] while extrinsic components are influences outside of you. When you think about it, it makes complete sense. If you are being badgered by a friend to join them in next year's ironman, this won't motivate you to do it in the way that an internal desire to do it would, or an external source that you personally subscribed to. If you're doing it only because your friend coerced you, then when the inevitable obstacles arise during the training phase, you won't have the necessary inner drive to carry on.

It's not often that you get inherent pleasure from partaking in a difficult task, so understanding the extrinsic component of motivation should give you some more flexibility in being able to manipulate your motivation levels to help achieve your objectives. A research study identified two types of extrinsic phenomena that represent the most freely initiated behaviour, way over on the right-hand side of our continuum:

1. Integrated regulation

2. Identified regulation

Integrated regulation – the belief that you engage in a particular behaviour because it is consistent with your identity or personal values – was found to be one of the most important determinants of exercise behaviour. You hear this when elite boxing athletes in interviews describe themselves as being 'fighters', a term which they aptly use to explain why they have decided to take up boxing.

This is closely followed by identified regulation, which refers to motivation deriving from behaviours that have personal significance or result in outcomes that you value highly. Someone may not glean any satisfaction from their job (intrinsic) or even see their identity as interwoven with their occupation (integrated), but the fact that they are able to work and provide for their family (identified) is significant enough to motivate them to continue that path. Unless you thoroughly enjoy the pleasures of your progressive behaviours, you will need mental toughness to keep you in the fight. Fortunately, this is something you can acquire through practice and action.

WORDS FROM COACH JAY

I was fourteen when I flew on my own from London Heathrow, which was an experience in itself, to attend basketball summer camp in the US. I was at the youngest end of the fourteen to eighteen age range for the cohort that year and was so much smaller than the other boys, who were gritty and resilient guys.

It was a tough camp, for many reasons, and I wasn't loving every minute of it like I thought I would before I arrived, but during those ten days I learned lessons about motivation and perseverance that have stayed with me.

Coach Jay was leading the charge and operations for the whole ten-day programme. The only way I can describe him was like the archetype of a military combatant. He was clean shaven with short hair, a chiselled jaw, piercing-blue eyes and muscles that resembled the shape and fullness of a perfectly formed cloud. He was a no-nonsense man.

The morning of the second day, Coach Jay sat us all down as he laid out the ground rules for the camp. There was a lot of call and response involved. He told us that when a drill, activity or instruction was explained to us by the coaches, they would ask us 'Is that clear?' to which we were to respond 'Crystal.'

If there was no clarity, then it would be re-explained until there was. 'What point is there,' he would say, 'in starting something you do not know how to do properly? First, get the instructions clear in your head.' Gulp.

Coach Jay said something profound that would be significant in determining how I was to approach not only the rest of camp, but also any challenge I wanted to overcome in life. His words, which echo just as loudly in my mind today as they did that morning, were:

'Your mind is your king.

Your body is your slave.

Your heart is your engine.

A king never listens to his slave.'

He was referencing the brutality of the coming days, that our bodies would want to give up on us because of the level of intensity that was coming, but we should settle in our minds that unless we were faced with serious injury, we wouldn't listen.

Was that clear? Crystal.

Below are some key techniques to augment the Cocoon Transformation principles and build your mental resilience.

Getting started

Getting started is simple enough to understand but not necessarily easy to do. It's simple because you will typically know what it is you need to do to get the ball rolling. There isn't much obscurity when it comes to beginning something you have on your to-do list; the reason it's often difficult to begin the process is because you are combatting all your internal inclinations to prolong your comfort. Comfort is an appealing idea until you equate it with idleness.

The key here is to remember that it won't always be this difficult every time you want to do the thing which you've set out in your mind to do. Eventually, you start to pick up momentum, which decreases the default resistance you previously had towards the task because you become accustomed to the idea that to be comfortable is to be idle, which gets you nowhere with regard to your goals.

Principle applied: Pick a date in your diary when you will start the process of working towards your goal, with the top three things on your agenda. Try not to be vague or ambiguous. If you are going to start learning a new language, then note down the books you intend to buy or the course you will enrol on. Try to be prescriptive in what exactly you are going to do.

Create milestones

If your challenge is a large one, it will take time to conquer it. Focusing on your ultimate aim can be overwhelming and paralyse you into not doing anything at all. The most successful people in the world purposefully implement a practice known as segmentation. It's a lot more glamorous for us to focus on the headline results, outcomes and successes, neglecting to appreciate the nuts and bolts of the processes that get us there. The irony is that those who are fixated on the glory tend never to come close to it, while those who obsess over the digestible steps usually achieve things that others are wide-eyed at.

Segmentation is about breaking down huge tasks into smaller, more digestible parts. If you've heard this before but haven't yet tried it, I would implore you to give it a real effort because, as cliché as it sounds, it is highly effective.

Principle applied: Just as you've scheduled time to start your process, diarise the next series of digestible parts of your overall vision that you can see from now. Expect this to evolve over time because, as you climb further up the mountain, you'll see just how far you've come and what steps will help you reach the next checkpoint.

Reframe for setbacks

Just when it seems like everything is going well with your plan, resources, accountability, health and any other thing that is contributing to your success, problems arise and knock your rhythm out of sync.

Things *will* go wrong at some stage. They always do and, frankly, I wouldn't have it any other way. If everyone had a straightforward and easy path to success, success wouldn't be what it is. The problems are needed to filter out the pretenders and to give you a deeper sense of accomplishment when you overcome them. Yes, you will have problems, but you mustn't let them derail you from the route to your destination. This is where your mettle is tested and forged, or tested and weakened.

One of the ways in which you can forge a tenacious spirit is through reframing – a technique that is used a lot in sales. Reframing is essentially discarding generic ideas, notions and beliefs used to present information, authority and status, and choosing your own frame to aid you in your objectives.

Principle applied: Actively rethink your interpretation of external events to suit your own objectives – in an ethical and honourable way, of course. For example, if your annual appraisal at work wasn't as good as you hoped, then instead of thinking of it as an attack on you, reframe it as your employer wanting to improve your performance towards undeniable levels excellence.

Visualise the journey and success

I will admit that I used to scoff at the purported benefits of visualisation. I thought it was hocus pocus and that it had no real part to play in advancing someone's mission. I used to think this way because I didn't really understand what it was. Like anything, I wanted to see some hard empirical evidence for these claims that the purveyors of this rhetoric could hang their hat on.

Then I started to learn that I'd conflated the concept of visualisation and its effects with other, poorly explained ideas. Visualisation has a neuroscientific basis and is an extremely powerful tool used by elite athletes. I was blown away when I came across a study that had conducted an experiment to determine strength gains induced by 'mental training'. The results were staggering. Although the study only looked at a tiny muscle on the outside of the little finger, the findings have significant ramifications for visualisation techniques. They found that the group of individuals who performed physical training exercises increased their little finger abductor strength by 53%, while those who did no physical exercise at all but performed exercises only in their minds increased their strength by 35%.[60]

Principle applied: Use visualisation techniques that engage all the senses to imagine specific details of the process applied and the success enjoyed. The aim is to make it feel as real as possible and use imagery that will encourage and uplift you, rather than frighten or panic you. You can choose how often you do this but make it regular and repetitive – ideally, you should do it every day. Eventually, it will become second nature for your mind to wander off into visualisations of your success.

PUNISHMENT FROM COACH JAY

Coach Jay had warned us right at the inception of camp to abide by the rules and have the right attitude in how we conducted ourselves. We were warned, I'll give him that.

He had an 'all for one, one for all' philosophy that he was instilling in us. The manifestation of this was that if any one of us intentionally violated the rules, the whole group of eighty boys would be punished severely for it. We only had three strikes to last us the whole ten days.

I wasn't at all bothered. We were all sensible and mature people, I thought. Why would we violate the rules when we were already at his mercy?

I remember sitting in my sub-group with Coach Andy on the third day when he told us that the boys already had two strikes. 'You have got to be joking me. When and how did this happen?' Clearly, rules had been broken by someone, but I didn't even bother to find out who – it wasn't up for appeal. The inevitable happened on the fifth day when Coach Jay had us all in the sports hall after a super intense evening of training. It was also pizza night, which we were all looking forward to.

'Gentlemen, you will go to the changing rooms and grab your things. We will then make our way back to the canteen hall where we will deal with our three strikes.'

The fear among us was tangible, and all I could do was prepare myself mentally to endure whatever our punishment would be, although I was fuming, having had nothing to do with the rule-breaking.

Once we got to the canteen hall, he told us all to find a space right under his line of sight so he could see all of us. Our punishment was that we had to do three push-ups... but each push-up lasted five minutes. With each push-up, Coach Jay instructed us to move closer to the ground by an inch or two, before moving further away from the ground by a few inches. This continued for five excruciatingly long minutes until he barked the golden word 'Down' to which we would reply 'Stronger', while going all the way down and fully extending our arms to finally complete the push-up.

If he wasn't satisfied with our efforts, he would stop and restart the timer. There was a lot of noise, a lot of pressure and a lot of pain. Boys much older than me were crying, it was that bad.

Once it was done, I didn't even want the pizza anymore, I just wanted to take my ball and go to bed. In retrospect, I can see how it was the lessons learned and physically arduous activity experienced at the camp that formed the early stages of my mental resilience.

Summary

The importance of mental toughness cannot be overstated. It is often assumed to exist only under extreme conditions, but this is not the case – we can all cultivate mental resilience in our everyday lives. Irrespective of the conditions, emotions are not a reliable guide for decision-making. The psychology behind staying motivated in circumstances that contradict your emotions can be explained by SDT. Pragmatically speaking, principles help you get started. Milestones define your next steps. Reframing prevents you giving up, and visualisation keeps you excited.

TEN
From Data To Greater: A Relational View

In this final chapter, we will explore the data showing how strength training positively impacts hormones, relationships and work-related stress. Here we'll also learn about the social aspect of health, an important component of wellbeing.

Progress monitoring

Research published by the American Psychological Association found that your chances of success increase in proportion to the level of progress monitoring that you engage in.[61] This shouldn't be surprising to you by now, given the methods we've discussed so far, but interestingly the study found that your chances increase even further when you report your progress publicly. When you share your progress with others, you make a public commitment to your goals, which increases your accountability – a factor we know is hugely important.

You probably know someone who has tried to work on something 'in secret' to spare themselves the embarrassment of failure. They mistakenly think that by keeping the pursuit of their goals private they can avoid any potential humiliation if it all goes belly-up, while still being able to enjoy the rewards that come from a public victory. This just isn't how the world works.

There are many reasons why efforts as a lone ranger often wane and success this way is rare, but the most compelling of these relates to relationships. At the most basic level, being able to communicate and share your ideas with another person will give you more clarity around what you are trying to do and, more importantly, *why* you are trying to do it.

At an even more substantive level, effective communication about your pursuits can deepen your relationships, providing you with expertise, insights and assistance to carry you to your next milestone. Accountability again comes into play here, because once you have invited someone to join your mission in offering you a helping hand, you will feel obliged at the very least to give it your best.

The power of collaborative efforts is incomprehensibly large, and every day lives change in small and big ways off the back of a single conversation with someone who knows just a bit more than the inquiring person does. Having information about our progress gives us something meaningful to talk about and gives us the privilege of accountability to others.

Now let's add to the equation.

Hormones

Humans are social creatures, and we generally care about what people think. We may not care about what *everyone* thinks about us, but we certainly care about how we are perceived by our closest family and friends. The more vibrant our outlook and brighter our countenance, the better able we are to foster the nourishing qualities that make our relationships with others stronger.

From a brain chemistry point of view, there are neurotransmitters and hormones that directly stimulate different parts of our brain and influence our emotions. Of course, everyday life doesn't consist only of events and experiences that bring about an uplift in our mood, even when we're with those we love. In fact, it's often easier to get frustrated with the people closest to us as we tend not to give them the benefit of the doubt and react in an impulsive way. On the positive side, though, the functions of the 'happy hormones' can help us enormously in our strength-training journey:

- Dopamine – the pleasure reinforcer
- Serotonin – the mood stabiliser
- Endorphins – the pain killer

Fortunately for you, all of these are released during your strength-training exercises and have transformative benefits for your mood and social interactions. The quiet and pleasurable craving you feel when you pack your gym bag knowing you are about to do a much-needed workout is due to the increased levels of dopamine released in your brain. The feeling that you get after a hard workout, when it feels like peaceful is your middle name, can be attributed to the release of serotonin. The easing of discomfort and/or clarity of mind you experience for hours after a gym session comes courtesy of endorphins.

It's easy to understand why you'd be compelled to keep detailed records when you build this awareness of how your body reacts to training. There are transcendent effects beyond the immediate, which can influence the seemingly most unrelated of things; you will certainly be able to see some of these correlations and effects in your life if you stick to the process. Overall, you'll be amazed at the effect that focusing on each component of this process and noticing the consequent benefits will have on shifting your disposition towards one that is a magnet for results.

A PLEASANT SURPRISE...

The fondness I had for my martial arts coach stirred up in me a desire to do something special for his thirtieth birthday, something that no one else would do. I also wanted to put my persistence and relationship management to the test, applying all I'd learned from my consistent training, enhanced mood and optimal behaviour patterns.

After giving it some thought, I decided that the best gift I could give him was a framed photo of his favourite UFC (Ultimate Fighting Championship) fighter in one of his most iconic moments, autographed and addressed to my coach with a personalised message. As if this wasn't audacious enough, I also wanted a video of the fighter addressing him by name and wishing him a happy birthday. Looking back, I think I must have been crazy, but I was also determined.

Where to even start? The fighter was still active and busy. He had a massive following, didn't manage any of his own social media channels and English wasn't his first language. I had no idea how I would make this happen and began to doubt whether it was even possible, just as I did when I started out on my journey to grow stronger than my friends.

I contacted dozens of gifting companies and people in the industry who I thought could help with my outlandish quest. If they bothered to reply at all, it was always the same: 'Sorry, we don't take those types of requests.' Eventually, I managed to find a small gifting company willing to help. I was to steer the direction of the operation while they were the hands and feet that executed it; it was a beautiful partnership but an extremely difficult project.

I'd lost count of how many dead-ends, refusals and discouraging moments we faced, but with the same principles I exercised during my strength training, I continued to persist and document our progress. Several months passed, my coach's birthday was seven weeks away and we weren't much closer to our goal. That was, until I had a stroke of genius. The calming effects of my strength training and progress monitoring led to an awakening and realisation of how I should apply inductive reasoning to the problem. In poetic fashion, once I actioned my part of the plan, the video arrived a few days before his birthday and the framed photo was delivered to my house on the day after his birthday, a class training day where I was able to present it to him in front of the rest of the guys.

He was speechless.

Your wellbeing matters. . . a lot

Decades of research have shown that you are more likely to have a heart attack on a Monday, between the hours of 6am and 9am, than at any other time in the week.[62] One study has even demonstrated that you are three times more likely to suffer a heart attack at 9am than you are at 11pm; the same is true for your risk of suffering a stroke.[63] It seems that people would – literally – rather die than face another week of work. Once your body decides that it has had enough, there is little that you can do to change its mind, but why wait until it gets to that point?

I find it mind-boggling how people treat their mind and personality as entities completely distinct from the body that houses them. It's alarming to see how many people abuse their bodies with alcohol, drugs and unhealthy lifestyle choices, as if there will be no consequences. Most people are precious about their phones and it often seems like they look after them better than they do their own bodies. You make sure your phone is always charged, locked and secure so that no one can tamper with it or access your private information. You always keep it close to you and do your best to protect it from falls with a case to minimise damage. If that fails and your phone is damaged in some way, it's likely covered by insurance enabling you to repair it or buy another one, vowing to treat it better than you did the last.

Is your body and wellbeing not more valuable than your phone?

The cost of stress

Work can be stressful, and stress can be extremely costly. Stress at work isn't in the best interests of you or your company, yet it has become the norm. In 2022, data curated from an employee experience platform showed that 89% of employees in the UK had experienced burnout in the last two years, with around a third suffering from physical and mental exhaustion.[64] A survey completed in 2018 also highlighted the extent of the issue when they shared their findings that 85% of UK adults feel stressed regularly and that they believed work was the second biggest cause of their stress, with money being the first.[65] Being signed-off work due to stress doesn't solve the problem, it only masks it for a while. Work-related stress is closely related to depression and anxiety which, according to the World Health Organization, costs the global economy up to $1 trillion a year in lost productivity – an incomprehensible number.[66] It's clear to see how stress is a problem not just for you, but for your employer as well – they need a happy and healthy workforce to function efficiently.

Knowing as we now do the benefits of physical exercise in general and strength training in particular for dealing with life's challenges, you can propose to your employer that they make certain accommodations for strength training or other exercise that could make a world of difference to their employees' stress levels, but you need to sound persuasive. To sound persuasive you need to *be* persuasive, so let's look at what research tells us there is to gain.

First up, is better job performance – a clear win for them. A UK study investigated occupations that are largely sedentary in nature and sought to find out the effects that exercising during the working day had on the work-related performance of 201 employees. Here are the results:[67]

- 79% reported better working relationships.

- 74% reported better workload management.

- 72% reported better time management.

- 57% improved in all three areas.

The level of energy and motivation to work observed on the days the participants did exercise was 41% higher than on the days they didn't. They were also 27% better at dealing calmly with workday stressors, 21% sharper in their concentration levels and 25% more likely to work without stopping to take unscheduled breaks. Now that is persuasive. By being able to explain to your employer why it's sensible for them to accommodate your strength training lifestyle and how this impacts their bottom line, they will be much more likely to take these considerations seriously. A friend of mine was able to incorporate his training around his working hours and became the top salesperson in his team. Kudos to him.

The second win is a personal one: reduced stress and burnout for yourself. A study conducted several years ago assessed the effectiveness of cardiovascular and resistance exercises as an intervention to combat occupational burnout. After just four weeks of exercise, participants experienced a multitude of benefits from resistance training, which had a notable effect on increasing their wellbeing and personal accomplishment, and reducing perceived stress.[68] The following year, another study revealed that improved muscular strength contributes to decreased neck and shoulder pain, leading to increased productivity. The employees in this study who spent most of their day sitting in an office or in front of a computer were less stressed and more energised when they were able to be physically active at their leisure.[69]

Do you see where I'm going with this? You shouldn't merely be allowed to strength train during your lunch breaks or at your leisure; you should be actively encouraged to do so by your boss, manager, colleagues and friends, because everybody wins in this equation. So compelling are the reasons for strength training that one doctor with over forty years' experience said, 'If you only have thirty minutes each week to exercise, you are much better off spending the time strength training than working on cardio.'[70]

You may well have a gym membership discount included in your benefits package, or an on-site gym if you're lucky. Despite this, the tone from the top is unlikely to reflect the tone in this book because most employers simply haven't embedded wellness and productivity into their strategy in the way presented here. If a gym membership isn't part of your benefits package, then it's high time you sat down with the person who can change that at your company – this is the twenty-first century after all.

Although it may seem counterintuitive, there is never any need to feel guilty or anxious that you're not getting your work done while you're exercising, because you are getting it done – strength training is an integral part of that work being done to a high standard. The data confirms this.

Summary

Progress monitoring is invaluable when it comes to orienting yourself to achieve your ambitions. Strength training comes with a constant flush of beneficial hormones, which help to stabilise your mood and benefit all types of relationships in various ways. This is particularly important for managing your general wellbeing and stress levels, which can become fatal if excessively neglected. There is profound empirical and anecdotal evidence to suggest that strength training at your leisure is supremely effective in managing work-related stress.

Conclusion

When you picked up this book, you may have had some fuzzy idea about the role strength training could play in your physical and mental well-being. Now, you have a thorough and comprehensive knowledge of the extent of the effects strength training has on how you live. You may not have noticed it beforehand, but you should now be able to see with fresh eyes how different your life could have been if you took strength training, and all the other principles and lessons that come with it, out of the equation. You also know that strength training is not enough on its own – you need to support it with information. *Your* information.

Behind all your highs, lows and everything in-between, is a body of knowledge that has been acquired, creating a path that can lead you to more success in the future. Unless you record the information that has got you to where you are, you can be sure that your progress will slow down, or stall entirely. Your training data is your compass, giving you clarity of vision, opening your eyes and showing you the direction of travel. This allows for full exploration of fundamental life changes and ultimately provides the key to a world of transformation.

It's tempting not to sweat the small stuff and think that this total, diligent commitment is not as necessary as I make it out to be, but it is. Consistent effort is an essential component of strength training if you want to experience more of the rewards it provides. You and I both know there is no room for laziness when building strength, but what if you learned that 20% of the effort you'd invested in your last workout had been effectively wasted? Compounded over many training sessions and many training years, the lost improvements become enormous. This 20% is in the seemingly small, trite details that you could be tempted to neglect.

It starts with getting twenty-twenty vision and crystal clarity on your objectives. You are the one who will be putting in the hard work, so it is you who must know what you want to achieve from it. Then, you need to make sure you are well equipped for battle. It will get hard at times, which is why many don't take the path you're on. Reluctance and half-heartedness won't lead to triumph. Those people who do things by halves haven't learned to apply this principle of being well equipped to their life outside of strength training. After reading this book, you won't be one of them.

The key lesson to retain, after clarity and resources, is accountability. No matter how strong-willed and talented you are, you can only ever get so far on your own. You need the help of others within a community with shared interests and goals to sharpen your clarity, further your knowledge and keep you on the path of consistent execution.

None of this happens without the underpinning of documentation. Keep an audit trail and observe the marked changes in you that your future self will thank you for. You need to get uncomfortable in your cocoon as that's the only way you will walk out of and beyond the weight room as a victor.

Notes

1   R Trussov, 'Here is how swimmers of all levels train (according to coaches)' (A3 Performance, 2020), www. a3performance.com/blogs/a3-performance/here-is-how-swimmers-of-all-levels-train-according-to-coaches, accessed 22 October 2022

2   'The law of marginal gains' (Sheridans, 2016), www. sheridansac.com.au/law-marginal-gains, accessed 22 October 2022

3   T Edwards, 'Rest between sets: What's right for me?' (Healthline, 11 June 2021), www.healthline.com/health/ fitness/rest-between-sets, accessed 15 March 2023; TJ Suchomel, S Nimphius et al, 'The importance of muscular strength: Training considerations', *Sports Medicine*, 48/4 (2018), 765–785, https://doi.org/10.1007/s40279-018-0862-z

4   J Clear, 'This coach improved every tiny thing by 1 percent and here's what happened' (James Clear, 2018), https:// jamesclear.com/marginal-gains, accessed 22 October 2022

5   JM Wilson, JP Loenneke, E Jo et al, 'The effects of endurance, strength, and power training on muscle fiber type shifting', *The Journal of Strength and Conditioning Research*, 26/6 (2012), 1724–1729, https://doi.org/10.1519/ JSC.0b013e318234eb6f

6   American College of Sports Medicine and American Heart Association, 'Exercise and acute cardiovascular events: Placing the risks into perspective', *Medicine and Science in Sports and Exercise*, 39/5 (2007), 886–897, https://doi.org/10.1249/mss.0b013e3180574e0e

7   SB Robertson, 'Weightlifting is better for the heart than cardio' (News-Medical.net, 9 July 2019), www.news-medical.net/amp/news/20190709/Weightlifting-is-better-for-the-heart-than-cardio.aspx, accessed 31 October 2022

8   AD Faigenbaum and GD Myer, 'Resistance training among young athletes: Safety, efficacy and injury prevention effects', *British Journal of Sports Medicine*, 44/1 (2010), 56–63, https://doi.org/10.1136/bjsm.2009.068098

9   C Ottinger, 'CNS fatigue' (The Muscle PhD, no date), https://themusclephd.com/cns-fatigue, accessed 27 October 2022

10 Y Liu, DC Lee, Y Li et al, 'Associations of resistance exercise with cardiovascular disease morbidity and mortality', *Medicine and Science in Sports and Exercise*, 51/3 (2019), 499, https://doi.org/10.1249/MSS.0000000000001822

11 JM Rijk, PR Roos, L Deckx et al, 'Prognostic value of handgrip strength in people aged 60 years and older: A systematic review and meta-analysis', *Geriatrics and Gerontology International*, 16/1 (2016), 5–20, https://doi.org/10.1111/ggi.12508

12 C Ottinger, 'Range of motion and growth' (The Muscle PhD, no date), https://themusclephd.com/range-of-motion-and-growth, accessed 4 November 2022

13 K Bloomquist, H Langberg, S Karlsen et al, 'Effect of range of motion in heavy load squatting on muscle and tendon adaptations', *European Journal of Applied Physiology*, 113/8 (2013), 2133–2142, https://doi.org/10.1007/s00421-013-2642-7; K Kubo, T Ikebukuro and H Yata, 'Effects of squat training with different depths on lower limb muscle volumes', *European Journal of Applied Physiology*, 119/9 (2019), 1933–1942, https://doi.org/10.1007/s00421-019-04181-y

14 RS Pinto, N Gomes, R Radaelli et al, 'Effect of range of motion on muscle strength and thickness', *The Journal of Strength and Conditioning Research*, 26/8 (2012), 2140–2145, https://doi.org/10.1519/jsc.0b013e31823a3b15

15 C Barakat, J Pearson, G Escalante et al, 'Body recomposition: Can trained individuals build muscle and lose fat at the same time?', *Strength and Conditioning Journal*, 42/5 (2020), 7–21, https://journals.lww.com/nsca-scj/fulltext/2020/10000/body_recomposition__can_trained_individuals_build.3.aspx; JE Donnelly, T Sharp, J Houmard et al, 'Muscle hypertrophy with large-scale weight loss and resistance training', *The American Journal of Clinical Nutrition*, 58/4 (1993), 561–565, https://doi.org/10.1093/ajcn/58.4.561; FB Del Vecchio, 'Body recomposition: Would it be possible to induce fat loss and muscle hypertrophy at the same time?', *Revista Brasileira de Cineantropometria e Desempenho Humano*, 24 (2022), e86265, https://doi.org/10.1590/1980-0037.2022v24e86265

16 C Ottinger, 'Body recomposition' (The Muscle PhD, no date), https://themusclephd.com/body-recomposition, accessed 4 November 2022

17 BR Gordon, CP McDowell, M Lyons et al, 'The effects of resistance exercise training on anxiety: A meta-analysis and meta-regression analysis of randomized controlled trials', *Sports Medicine*, 47/12 (2017), 2521–2532, https://doi.org/10.1007/s40279-017-0769-0

18 C Pickering and J Kiely, 'Do non-responders to exercise exist – and if so, what should we do about them?' *Sports Medicine*, 49/1 (2019), 1–7, https://doi.org/10.1007/s40279-018-01041-1

19 J Antonio, A Ellerbroek, T Silver et al, 'A high protein diet (3.4g/kg/d) combined with a heavy resistance training program improves body composition in healthy trained men and women – a follow-up investigation', *Journal of the International Society of Sports Nutrition*, 12/1 (2015), 39, https://doi.org/10.1186/s12970-015-0100-0; BI Campbell, D Aguilar, L Conlin et al, 'Effects of high versus low protein intake on body composition and maximal strength in aspiring female physique athletes engaging in an 8-week resistance training program', *International Journal of Sport Nutrition and Exercise Metabolism*, 28/6 (2018), 580–585, https://doi.org/10.1123/ijsnem.2017-0389; PJ Cribb, AD Williams, MF Carey et al, 'The effect of whey isolate and resistance training on strength, body composition, and plasma glutamine', *International Journal of Sport Nutrition*

and Exercise Metabolism, 16/5 (2006), 494–509, https://doi.org/10.1123/ijsnem.16.5.494

20 PJ Arciero, MJ Ormsbee, CL Gentile et al, 'Increased protein intake and meal frequency reduces abdominal fat during energy balance and energy deficit', *Obesity*, 21/7 (2013), 1357–1366, https://doi.org/10.1002/oby.20296; C Barakat, J Pearson, G Escalante et al, 'Body recomposition: Can trained individuals build muscle and lose fat at the same time?', *Strength and Conditioning Journal*, 42/5 (2020), 7–21, https://doi.org/10.1519/SSC.0000000000000584

21 See, for example, J Axe, *Keto Diet Cookbook: 125+ delicious recipes to lose weight, balance hormones, boost brain health, and reverse disease* (Little Brown Spark, 2019)

22 P Bazire, 'Introduction to the Mediterranean diet' (PDF shared with the author) (Bazire Medical Weight Management, 1 July 2022)

23 JM McNamara, RL Swalm, DJ Stearne et al, 'Online weight training', *The Journal of Strength and Conditioning Research*, 22/4 (2008), 1164–1168, https://doi.org/10.1519/JSC.0b013e31816eb4e0

24 E Sundstrup, MD Jakobsen, CH Andersen et al, 'Muscle activation strategies during strength training with heavy loading vs. repetitions to failure', *The Journal of Strength and Conditioning Research*, 26/7 (2012), 1897–1903, https://doi.org/10.1519/JSC.0b013e318239c38e

25 CJ Mitchell, TA Churchward-Venne, DW West et al, 'Resistance exercise load does not determine training-mediated hypertrophic gains in young men', *Journal of Applied Physiology*, 113/1 (2012), 71–77, https://doi.org/10.1152/japplphysiol.00307.2012

26 PW Marshall, M McEwen and DW Robbins, 'Strength and neuromuscular adaptation following one, four, and eight sets of high-intensity resistance exercise in trained males', *European Journal of Applied Physiology*, 111/12 (2011), 3007–3016, https://doi.org/10.1007/s00421-011-1944-x

27 M Jovanovic and EP Flanagan, 'Research applications of velocity-based strength training', *Journal of Australian Strength and Conditioning*, 21/1 (2014), 58–69, www.researchgate.net/profile/Eamonn-Flanagan/publication/265227430_Researched_Applications_of_Velocity_Based_Strength_Training/links/543690a60cf2dc341db35e79/Researched-

Applications-of-Velocity-Based-Strength-Training.pdf, accessed 31 March 2023

28 MA Goolsby, 'Overtraining: What it is, symptoms and recovery' (Hospital for Special Surgery, 16 August 2021), www.hss.edu/article_overtraining.asp, accessed 7 November 2022

29 D Pacheco, 'Why do we need sleep?' (Sleep Foundation, 10 August 2022), www.sleepfoundation.org/how-sleep-works/why-do-we-need-sleep, accessed 7 November 2022

30 J Born, R Pietrowsky, P Pauschinger et al, 'Secretion of growth hormone during slow-wave sleep deprivation', *European Journal of Endocrinology*, 116/3 (1987), S60–S61, https://doi.org/10.1530/acta.0.114S060

31 T Sözen, L Özışık and NC Başaran, 'An overview and management of osteoporosis', *European Journal of Rheumatology*, 4/1 (2017), 46–56, https://doi.org/10.5152/eurjrheum.2016.048

32 S Khosla, MJ Oursler and DG Monroe, 'Estrogen and the skeleton', *Trends in Endocrinology and Metabolism*, 23/11 (2012), 576–581, https://doi.org/10.1016/j.tem.2012.03.008

33 X Zhang, KW Man, GHY Li et al, 'Osteoporosis is a novel risk factor of infections and sepsis: A cohort study', *eClinicalMedicine*, 49 (2022), 101488, https://doi.org/10.1016/j.eclinm.2022.101488

34 YC Tseng, CC Tsai, JH Cheng et al, 'Recognizing the peak bone mass (age 30) as a cutoff point to achieve the success of orthodontic implants', *Odontology*, 108/3 (2020), 503–510, https://doi.org/10.1007/s10266-019-00476-w

35 H Wilson and D Finch, 'Unemployment and mental health' (The Health Foundation, 2021), www.health.org.uk/sites/default/files/2021-04/2021, accessed 7 November 2022

36 S Frye, 'Callus | dermatology', *Encyclopædia Britannica* (20 July 1998), www.britannica.com/science/callus-dermatology, accessed 9 November 2022

37 E Volpi, R Nazemi and S Fujita, 'Muscle tissue changes with aging', *Current opinion in Clinical Nutrition and Metabolic Care*, 7/4 (2004), 405–410, https://doi.org/10.1097/01.mco.0000134362.76653.b2

38 J Choi, 'How to master the art of to-do lists by understanding why they fail', *I Done This Blog* (23 February 2021), http://blog.idonethis.com/how-to-master-the-art-of-to-do-lists, accessed 10 November 2022

39   JB Lauersen, TE Andersen and LB Andersen, 'Strength
     training as superior, dose-dependent and safe prevention
     of acute and overuse sports injuries: A systematic review,
     qualitative analysis and meta-analysis', *British Journal
     of Sports Medicine*, 52/24 (2018), 1557–1563, https://doi.
     org/10.1136/bjsports-2018-099078

40   K Valluzzi, 'People don't keep records of their workouts'
     (Trainerize.me, 3 April 2017), www.trainerize.me/
     articles/peoplep-dont-keep-records-workouts, accessed 11
     November 2022

41   DA Bonilla, LA Cardozo, JM Vélez-Gutiérrez et al,
     'Exercise selection and common injuries in fitness
     centers: A systematic integrative review and practical
     recommendations', *International Journal of Environmental
     Research and Public Health*, 19/19 (2022), 12710, https://doi.
     org/10.3390/ijerph191912710

42   NW Hudson and RC Fraley, 'Do people's desires to change
     their personality traits vary with age? An examination of
     trait change goals across adulthood', *Social Psychological
     and Personality Science*, 7/8 (2016), 847–856, https://doi.
     org/10.1177/1948550616657598; M Stieger, S Wepfer, D
     Rüegger et al, 'Becoming more conscientious or more open
     to experience? Effects of a two-week smartphone-based
     intervention for personality change', *European Journal of
     Personality*, 34/3 (2020), 345–366, https://doi.org/10.1002/
     per.2267

43   O Khazan, 'I gave myself three months to change my
     personality', *The Atlantic* (10 February 2022), www.theatlantic.
     com/magazine/archive/2022/03/how-to-change-your-
     personality-happiness/621306, accessed 14 November 2022

44   BW Roberts, J Luo, DA Briley et al, 'A systematic review of
     personality trait change through intervention', *Psychological
     Bulletin*, 143/2 (2017), 117–141, https://doi.org/10.1037/
     bul0000088

45   NW Hudson and RC Fraley, 'Volitional personality trait
     change: Can people choose to change their personality
     traits?', *Journal of Personality and Social Psychology*, 109/3
     (2015), 490–507, https://doi.org/10.1037/pspp0000021

46   'Conscientiousness: A "big five" personality trait',
     Psychologist World (no date), www.psychologistworld.com/
     influence-personality/conscientiousness-personality-trait,
     accessed 17 February 2023

47 A Doherty and A Forés Miravalles, `Physical activity and cognition: Inseparable in the classroom', *Frontiers in Education*, 4/105 (2019), https://doi.org/10.3389/feduc.2019.00105

48 JK Ma, L Le Mare and BJ Gurd, 'Four minutes of in-class high-intensity interval activity improves selective attention in 9- to 11-year olds', *Applied Physiology, Nutrition, and Metabolism*, 40/3 (2015), 238–244, https://doi.org/10.1139/apnm-2014-0309

49 DE Conroy and AJ Elliot, 'Fear of failure and achievement goals in sport: Addressing the issue of the chicken and the egg', *Anxiety, Stress, and Coping*, 17/3 (2004), 271–285, https://doi.org/10.1080/1061580042000191642

50 S Gardner and D Albee, 'Study focuses on strategies for achieving goals, resolutions', press release, *Dominican Scholar* (2015), 266, https://scholar.dominican.edu/news-releases/266, accessed 31 March 2023

51 M Forleo, 'Self-made millionaire: The simple strategy that helped increase my odds of success by 42%' (CNBC, 13 September 2019), www.cnbc.com/2019/09/13/self-made-millionaire-how-to-increase-your-odds-of-success-by-42-percent-marie-forleo.html, accessed 18 February 2023

52 G Gill, 'Mental toughness' (BelievePerform, no date), https://believeperform.com/mental-toughness, accessed 18 November 2022

53 K Dilanian and C Kube, 'Navy SEAL candidate dies, second hospitalized following "Hell Week" training', *NBC News* (5 February 2022), www.nbcnews.com/news/navy-seal-candidate-dies-second-hospitalized-hell-week-training-rcna15036, accessed 18 November 2022

54 D Trampe, J Quoidbach and M Taquet, 'Emotions in everyday life', *PLOS ONE*, 10/12 (2015), e0145450, https://doi.org/10.1371/journal.pone.0145450

55 'What is anxiety?' (Mental Health UK, 2019), https://mentalhealth-uk.org/help-and-information/conditions/anxiety-disorders/what-is-anxiety, accessed 7 November 2022

56 'People seeking help: Statistics' (Mental Health Foundation, no date), www.mentalhealth.org.uk/explore-mental-health/mental-health-statistics/people-seeking-help-statistics, accessed 7 November 2022

57 'Coronavirus and depression in adults, Great Britain' (Office for National Statistics, 1 October 2021), www.ons.

gov.uk/peoplepopulationandcommunity/wellbeing/
articles/coronavirusanddepressioninadultsgreatbritain/
julytoaugust2021#prevalence-of-depressive-symptoms-
over-time, accessed 7 November 2022

58 PJ O'Connor, MP Herring and A Caravalho, 'Mental health
benefits of strength training in adults', *American Journal
of Lifestyle Medicine*, 4/5 (2010), 377–396, https://doi.
org/10.1177/1559827610368771

59 LR Duncan, CR Hall, PM Wilson et al, 'Exercise motivation:
A cross-sectional analysis examining its relationships with
frequency, intensity, and duration of exercise', *International
Journal of Behavioral Nutrition and Physical Activity*, 7 (2010),
article 7, https://doi.org/10.1186/1479-5868-7-7

60 VK Ranganathan, V Siemionow, JZ Liu et al, 'From mental
power to muscle power – gaining strength by using the
mind', *Neuropsychologia*, 42/7 (2004), 944–956, https://doi.
org/10.1016/j.neuropsychologia.2003.11.018

61 B Harkin, TL Webb, BP Chang et al, 'Does monitoring goal
progress promote goal attainment? A meta-analysis of the
experimental evidence', *Psychological Bulletin*, 142/2 (2016),
198–229, https://doi.org/10.1037/bul0000025

62 MC Cohen, KM Rohtla, CE Lavery et al, 'Meta-analysis
of the morning excess of acute myocardial infarction
and sudden cardiac death', *The American Journal of
Cardiology*, 79/11 (1997), 1512–1516, https://doi.
org/10.1016/s0002-9149(97)00181-1; DR Witte, DE Grobbee,
ML Bots et al, 'A meta-analysis of excess cardiac mortality
on Monday', *European Journal of Epidemiology*, 20/5
(2005), 401–406, https://doi.org/10.1007/s10654-004-
8783-6; JE Muller and GH Tofler, 'Circadian variation
and cardiovascular disease', *New England Journal
of Medicine*, 325/14 (1991), 1038–1039, https://doi.
org/10.1056/NEJM199110033251410

63 H Ostrem, 'If you're going to have a stroke or STEMI,
here's when it might happen!' (Pulsara, 10 December
2015), www.pulsara.com/blog/if-youre-going-to-have-
a-stroke-or-stemi-heres-when-it-might-happen, accessed
23 November 2022; M Ahmed, 'Predicting a heart
attack – what are the chances?' (MyHeart, 23 January
2015), https://myheart.net/articles/predict-heart-
attack, accessed 23 November 2022; JE Muller and GH
Tofler, 'Circadian variation and cardiovascular disease',

New England Journal of Medicine, 325/14 (1991), 1038–1039, https://doi.org/10.1056/NEJM199110033251410

64 LumApps, 'How to boost employee sentiment in 2022' (LumApps, 29 January 2022), www.lumapps.com/webinars/how-to-boost-employee-sentiment-in-2022, accessed 23 November 2022

65 'Great Britain and stress – how bad is it and why is it happening?' (Forth, 2018), www.forthwithlife.co.uk/blog/great-britain-and-stress, accessed 31 March 2023

66 World Health Organization, 'Mental health at work' (WHO, 28 September 2022), www.who.int/news-room/fact-sheets/detail/mental-health-at-work, accessed 23 November 2022.

67 JC Coulson, J McKenna and M Field, 'Exercising at work and self-reported work performance', *International Journal of Workplace Health Management*, 1/3 (2008), 176–197, https://doi.org/10.1108/17538350810926534

68 RJ Bretland and EB Thorsteinsson, 'Reducing workplace burnout: The relative benefits of cardiovascular and resistance exercise', *PeerJ*, 3 (2015), e891, https://doi.org/10.7717/peerj.891; 'Can resistance training improve well-being at work?' (Ddrobotec, no date), https://ddrobotec.com/can-resistance-training-improve-well-being-at-work, accessed 23 November 2022.

69 G Sjøgaard, JR Christensen, JB Justesen et al, 'Exercise is more than medicine: The working age population's well-being and productivity', *Journal of Sport and Health Science*, 5/2 (2016), 159–165, https://doi.org/10.1016/j.jshs.2016.04.004

70 D Tesch, 'Better strength leads to better job performance', *HealthPartners Blog* (15 August 2019), www.healthpartners.com/blog/better-strength-leads-to-better-job-performance, accessed 23 November 2022

Acknowledgements

I'd like to thank my dear wife, Marilyn. Your direct and ancillary support of my writing journey has been deeply encouraging and gracefully forbearing – I love you.

A huge thank you to Michele Rosso, Dan Thomas, Roy Garcia-Singh, Temi Akomolafe and KC Bulaon.

All of your stories in their entirety have reinforced in my mind why it was necessary to write this book.

Thank you, Ioannis Souriadakis, Marios Kamperis and David Strömbäck, for supporting this book and allowing me the time to focus on our philosophy of creating more victors.

This book would not have been what it is without the constructive feedback of my beta readers Josh Hurley, Michael Oduyela, Michael Simmons and Nathan Sinclair.

I'd also like to extend my heartfelt gratitude to Anke Ueberberg, Kathleen Steeden and Abi Willford for their intensive editorial work on my manuscript.

Lastly, there would be no book at all if Lucy McCarraher hadn't encouraged me before the first word was inscribed. I'm truly grateful.